DISCOVER THE

SYNERGETICS

WAY TO COMPLETE FITNESS
AND WELL-BEING!

Far more than a program of physical exercise, *Synergetics* is a *whole life fitness plan*. Its root word, *synergy*, means a combined action whose total effect is greater than the sum of the individual actions. Most exercise programs isolate muscle groups and "spot"-exercise them—working on just a few muscles at a time. With Synergetics, your whole body works in harmony for beauty, strength, and well-being.

The system is so easy and effective that it can be used as a conditioning program by people of any age. *Without* hours in the gym, expensive equipment, pain or strain, you can take the first best step to lifetime fitness, with *Synergetics!*

"A fascinating movement package which promises to entice preschoolers and octogenarians alike to pivot, dip, and smile their way to better health."

—Bryant A. Stamford, Ph.D.
Professor and Director,
University of Louisville Health Promotion Center

"As a surgeon, I found that my hands became a lot stronger after using Synergetics, which was an unexpected benefit. I find myself doing these exercises on the elevators and in my office in between patients. . . . For those people who have been away from exercise for years, Synergetics is a safe way to get started again without fear of complications to one's health."

—William M. Moses, M.D.

"This unique approach is overdue. It is safe, effective, and rational exercise you can really enjoy. This program will invigorate you in a way you never thought possible. . . . I recommend this program without reservation. Synergetics is super."

—Craig A. Mueller, D.C.

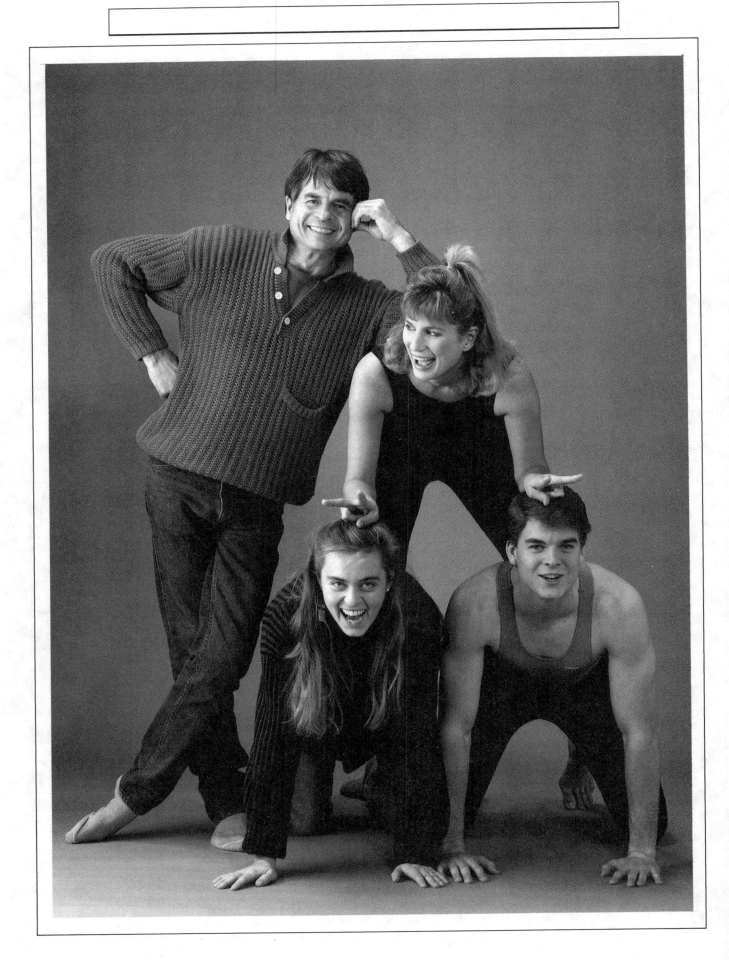

SYNERGETICS

YOUR WHOLE LIFE FITNESS PLAN

Taylor and Joanna Hay

6/22/06

SUSAN!

Enjoy in Good Health!

Taylor and Joanna

POCKET BOOKS

New York   London   Toronto   Sydney   Tokyo   Singapore

An *Original* publication of POCKET BOOKS

POCKET BOOKS, a division of Simon & Schuster Inc.
1230 Avenue of the Americas, New York, NY 10020

Copyright © 1990 by You Can Be A Classic, Inc.
Cover photo © 1990 by Mort Engel
Book design by Richard Oriolo

ISBN: 0-671-67397-1

First Pocket Books trade paperback printing February 1990

10 9 8 7 6 5 4 3

POCKET and colophon are registered trademarks of Simon & Schuster Inc.

Printed in the U.S.A.

ACKNOWLEDGMENTS

Among the many people who have helped and encouraged us to keep working on this rewarding project, we owe special thanks to two friends: Reavis Boyd, for his work to see that this book was written, and Bill Scheutze who unselfishly shared his time and experience. And thanks to John Hay and Mary Belle for their love and support.

Our love and thanks to our models, Diane Hay Beckman and Williams Hay, and to Diane's children, Whit, Lindley, Hillary, and Beau Taylor.

Thanks to our editors, Elaine Pfefferblit and Laura Cronin, who gave us an extra special share of their time and energy; to our photographers, Mike Parker of the Paul Schultz Company and Mort and Sydell Engel; and our agent, Richard Curtis. We would also like to acknowledge the special contribution of the people at Jeté Bodywear and Hind Athletic Wear who saw to it that we were outfitted for the 1990s.

To Taylor III, Shelley, Diane, Ambie, Robert,
Douglas, Elisabeth, and Williams

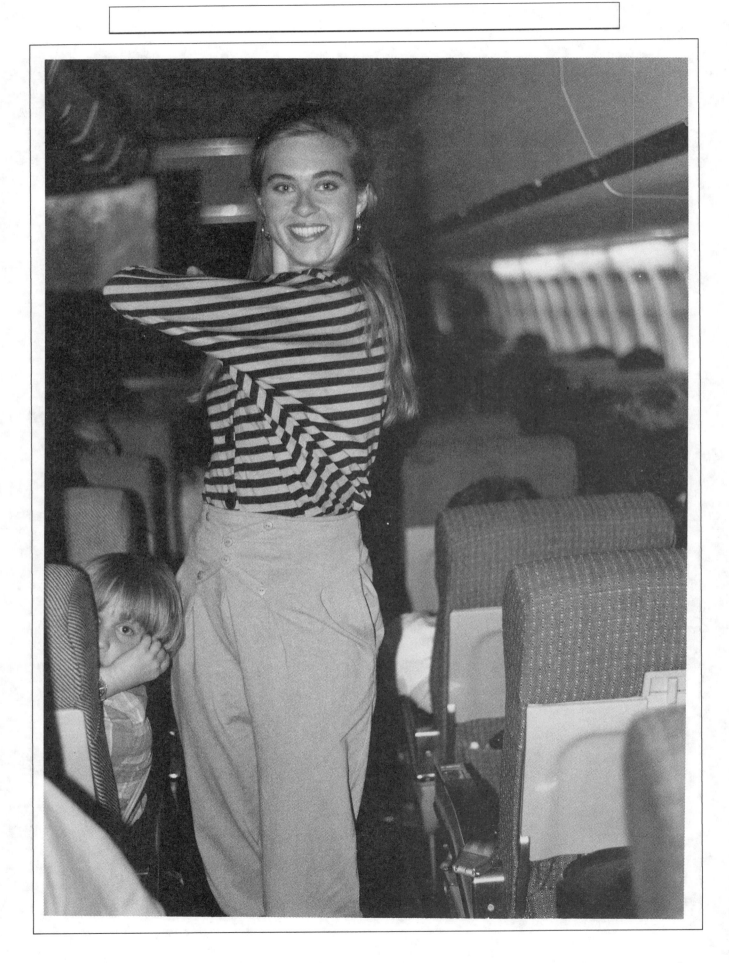

CONTENTS

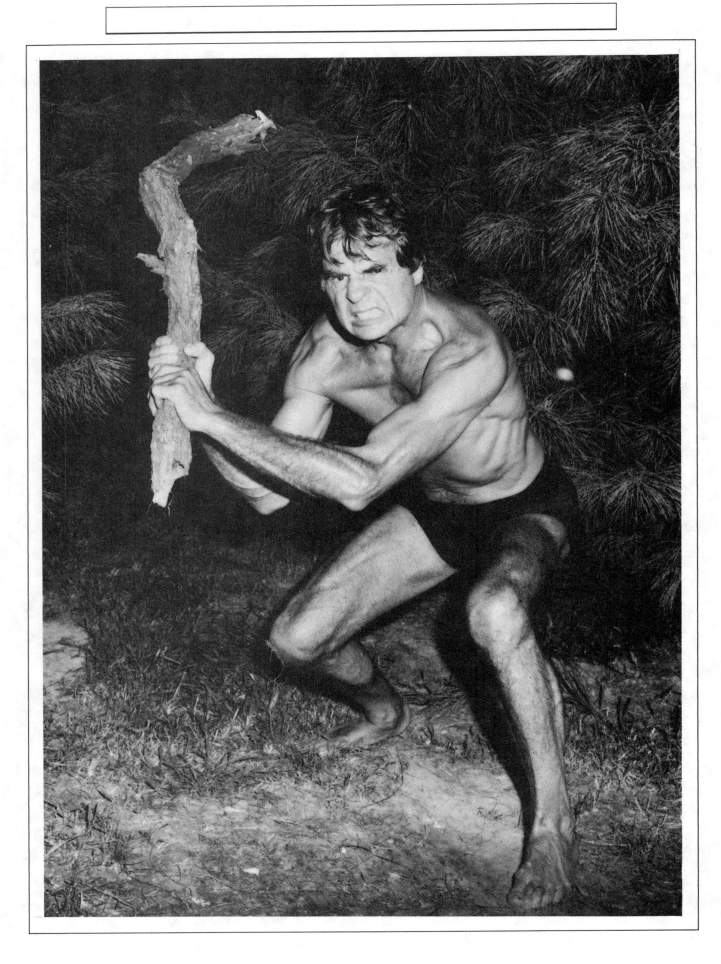

FOREWORD

YOUR WHOLE LIFE
FITNESS PLAN

In prehistoric times, human beings spent almost every waking moment concentrating on survival. We hunted for wild game on foot, we gathered fruits, nuts, and vegetables by hand, and drank from glacier-fed streams. Our bodies became compatible with the climate and the foods of our region. We developed to accommodate the physical demands of hunting and gathering. Our brains grew enormously and we began to use our hands to make tools and weapons. Our bodies became tall, strong, and well coordinated, more like present-day Olympic athletes—so strong that we were able to track animals for miles, make the kill, and then carry the meat back to our shelters. Our greatest enemies were famine, wild beasts, earthquakes, and volcanic eruptions. In spite of these physical challenges, we have survived to the dawn of the twenty-first century.

So, here we are, still in possession of the same bodies and the same physical abilities that enabled our species to survive for millions of years. That's the good news. The bad news is that many of us are not feeding and exercising our bodies in a manner that is natural to them; we are aging too quickly with ever-shortening healthspans. Our bodies still need the exercise that our ancestors got when they had to hunt and gather every day for survival, and we still need the foods that were essential to our evolution over millions of years. In short, our bodies need more daily physical exercise, fresh, unprocessed foods, and pure water than they get now.

Since very few of us have the desire to "go back to nature" and live off the land, our next best option is to figure out how we can have the best of both worlds—the conveniences of today, and the healthy, active lifestyle of our prehistoric past. We can't control all of the hazards that surround us, but we do have the ability to build a powerful body and immune system capable of withstanding the many environmental shocks we're continually subjected to. By supercharging our bodies every day with invigorating exercises, highly nutritious foods, and pure water, we can add many healthy years to our lives.

Synergetics is your guide to the creation of a personal Whole Life Fitness Plan for thriving in an often hostile world—a world which is, nevertheless, filled with excitement, challenge, and beauty.

INTRODUCTION

Millions of people are working out every day with jogging, aerobics, weights, and other exercise programs, but millions more don't have the desire, physical ability, or time to go through such strenuous, time-consuming workouts. So, many people are just sitting on the sidelines, watching the dedicated few get in shape, and wishing they could find a simple way to take care of themselves.

All of my life I have been searching for ways to keep my body healthy. I have experimented with many different exercises at different times in my life. As a young boy I did Charles Atlas's Dynamic Tension and lifted rusty barbells in the basement of a YMCA. In college I trained for football by sprinting up and down the field, with a lot of weight lifting and high-speed calisthenics mixed in. Running a couple of miles in a park started off my mornings for twenty-five years. I supplemented my run with isometrics, a rowing machine, free weights, deep knee bends, chins, push-ups, and sit-ups. I got my money's worth from my lifetime membership at the neighborhood health club. I pulled and pushed on the first Universal weight machines, and flexed and toned with Nautilus. I tried aerobics. I owned a rebounder, and experimented with gravity exercises while hanging upside down. I wore out several extra-heavy rubber exercise straps, and climbed up and down a rope hanging from a tree limb in my backyard. Whenever I could, I played touch football and pickup basketball. My sister introduced me to Tai Chi Ch'uan and Aikido, and I took some Yoga classes to see what they were like. Yoga was relaxing, but my body ached for action!

I loved the action of sports. I loved the shiny exercise equipment, the companionship of fellow exercisers, the mirrors, the steam room, the whirlpool, the tanning booth, the muscles, the sweat. I loved running in the park, chinning from the basement rafters. To me, strenuous physical exercise was a tranquilizer, an energizer, a temporary way out of the daily stress of my very stressful life. Back then I would have laughed if someone had told me that I was permanently injuring my body with exercise.

By the time I was fifty, my joints were worn out. I had overdone the exercises. I had overextended my body. I had unknowingly weakened myself, little by little, until I had to give up altogether on the sports and exercises that I loved. After a few months of not exercising, I lost all of the muscle tone and endurance I had worked so hard to keep up over the years. It made me tired just to carry a couple of bags of groceries up the steps to my kitchen. My body began to sag under the extra pounds I gained, and my face began to look old and tired. One night I looked in a full-length mirror and felt that I had aged ten years in just a few months.

A PROFILE OF PAIN

It never entered my mind that I could injure myself with the very exercises that were supposed to keep me in shape. What I didn't know is that the cartilage which padded my joints had no way of signaling me that I was destroying it. Since the cartilage had no nerve endings or feeling, I unknowingly abused it for years with joint-shocking exercises until it cracked, granulated, and became a useless mass of painful scar tissue.

For many years I took body-degenerating cortisone shots in both shoulders, both knees, and my Achilles' tendons to relieve excruciating pain.

THE DISCOVERY

In desperation I went back to my health club and tried to lift weights again. I got a hernia the first week and had to have an operation. When I got out of the hospital, I drove to a deserted beach on the coast of North Carolina, rented a little shack on stilts overlooking the sand dunes, and just sat there, trying to heal. After a few days I began experimenting with different types of light exercises—hoping to discover some motions that wouldn't hurt my already badly damaged body. I tried every exercise imaginable—bending, dancing, prancing, stretching—but none of them seemed right, and most of them hurt.

Then in the middle of one night my eyes popped open with a flash of an idea—a brainstorm! I quickly got up, turned on a dim light, and began doing motions that I had never done before in my life. I knew right away that I was moving in a way that felt good and didn't hurt! I spent the rest of the night standing on my favorite sand dune, experimenting with my newfound motions until the sun came up sparkling over the rim of the ocean. Within a few days I had the beginnings of a new body. I had stumbled upon a new way to exercise.

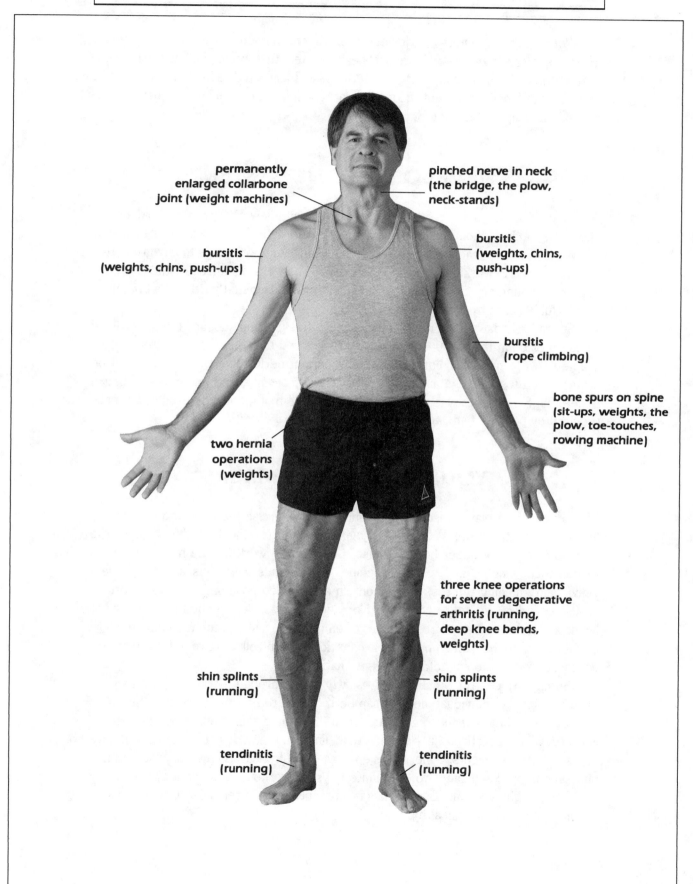

permanently
enlarged collarbone
joint (weight machines)

pinched nerve in neck
(the bridge, the plow,
neck-stands)

bursitis
(weights, chins, push-ups)

bursitis
(weights, chins,
push-ups)

bursitis
(rope climbing)

bone spurs on spine
(sit-ups, weights, the
plow, toe-touches,
rowing machine)

two hernia
operations
(weights)

three knee operations
for severe degenerative
arthritis (running,
deep knee bends,
weights)

shin splints
(running)

shin splints
(running)

tendinitis
(running)

tendinitis
(running)

With enormous energy, I devoted every spare moment of the next nine years to developing an enjoyable and practical health system that would give me the benefits of all of the exercises I had ever done in the past. I learned that I didn't need a lot of time, a lot of fancy equipment, a lot of sweat, and a lot of painful injuries just to keep my body in shape—I needed Synergetics.

DEVELOPING THE SYSTEM

I studied exercise books, read medical papers, health newsletters, and books on the physiology and psychology of the human body. I consulted with physicians. I traveled all over my region, teaching Synergetics on evenings and weekends to any group that was interested in working with me. Each year I was welcomed back by these groups of people, young and old—all enthusiastic and many claiming that they had received wonderful benefits from Synergetics.

It gradually dawned on me that Synergetics was truly unique, and that it occupied a special place in the world of exercise. I discovered that the motions automatically adapted to the needs or limitations of the person performing them, and could be programmed to challenge any individual's strength, agility, and endurance. I began to see that Synergetics was so easy and so effective that it could be used as a fitness program by people of any age and almost any physical condition.

YOUR BODY REMEMBERS

Most exercises isolate muscle groups and "spot" exercise them—working on just a few muscles at a time. Walking and jogging emphasize the legs, but neglect the development of the upper body because there is little work for the hands and arms to do. Free weights and weight machines isolate muscle groups and work them individually, holding the rest of the body in a semifixed position. Strenuous aerobic programs utilize the entire body but, like jogging, pay little attention to working the hands and arms with any force, and are often done too fast and too randomly to allow the motions to be remembered, or consciously controlled—two things that are necessary for developing total body coordination.

Total body control is achieved by slowly going through motions with a focused mind so that the individual motions can be remembered by the brain and the body. New or learned motions become ingrained in the brain circuitry only when movement is repeated and practiced, just as healthy feelings and attitudes are learned when we repeat positive thoughts. Synergetics employs this physical and mental programming phenomena by combining two 12-minute physical workout sessions a day with two positive thought sessions. Synergetics is a practical way to remind your body to stay physically and mentally healthy.

DON'T BE HYPNOTIZED BY YOUR AGE!

It may sound corny, but my mother gave me the best advice of my life. She leaned over to me at a Thanksgiving dinner and whispered, "Son, don't *ever* be hypnotized by your age." Because of her advice, I am very conscious of the age stereotypes that are presented to me in magazines, cartoons, and television programs. I have practiced not being affected by people who use age clichés like "Act your age!," or "Slow down, you're not as young as you used to be."

Years ago, my great-great-grandfather, Colonel E. H. Taylor, Jr., lay near death in his home in Frankfort, Kentucky. His business was in collapse, and his house was being foreclosed on. Two doctors stood in the upstairs hall outside his bedroom whispering to each other. "Too bad the old colonel is dying," said one. "Yes, and it's unfortunate that he is dying broke," the other replied. Colonel Taylor overheard their conversation. His eyes snapped open, he leapt out of bed, ran into the hall in his flowing nightshirt, and chased the surprised doctors down the stairs and out the front door. Shaking his fist at their retreating coattails, he bellowed, "I'm not dying, and I'll be damned if I'll die broke!" He didn't. He lived twenty-three more years, and died at the age of ninety-three after founding several whiskey distilleries. He left a fortune to his family, a fine bourbon whiskey in his memory (Old Taylor Kentucky Straight Bourbon), and a legacy in courage and determination for anyone who wants to follow his example.

Regardless of your past, you can have a perfect future. Never give up on yourself or your life. Whether you are very young or very old, it makes no difference. With Synergetics, you can take the first best step to perfecting your own life. You can be sure that your body, mind, and spirit are whole and you can enjoy the graces that shower on you each and every day.

WE AREN'T FAKING

The wild claims of advertisers can make a cynic out of a saint, so we thought that we had better tell you right off that we aren't faking about what Synergetics has done for us. Some people suspect that we eat like rabbits—a leaf of lettuce, a pinch of sprouts, and a few slivers of carrots. Some think that we work out with special machines or weights to keep our shapes. The truth is that we eat three good meals a day and exercise with Synergetics.

It's also true that sometimes we get lazy and don't exercise, and sometimes we dive into junk food. With Synergetics, these lapses never last very long. When we stop exercising, we miss the energy that we know we can get from our twice-a-day,

12-minute workouts. When we binge on junk food, we begin to miss the feeling of well-being we know comes from wholesome, natural food.

Our bodies never fake how they feel, so we give them what they ask for—fewer lapses into inactivity and unhealthy eating, and more energizing Synergetics motion.

When I first got into a Synergetics routine I was thirty pounds heavier than I am now. Twelve minutes in the morning and twelve minutes in the evening steadily made the weight drop off and I went from 151 pounds to 121 pounds in seven months— and I've kept that weight.

Joanna

SYNERGETICS

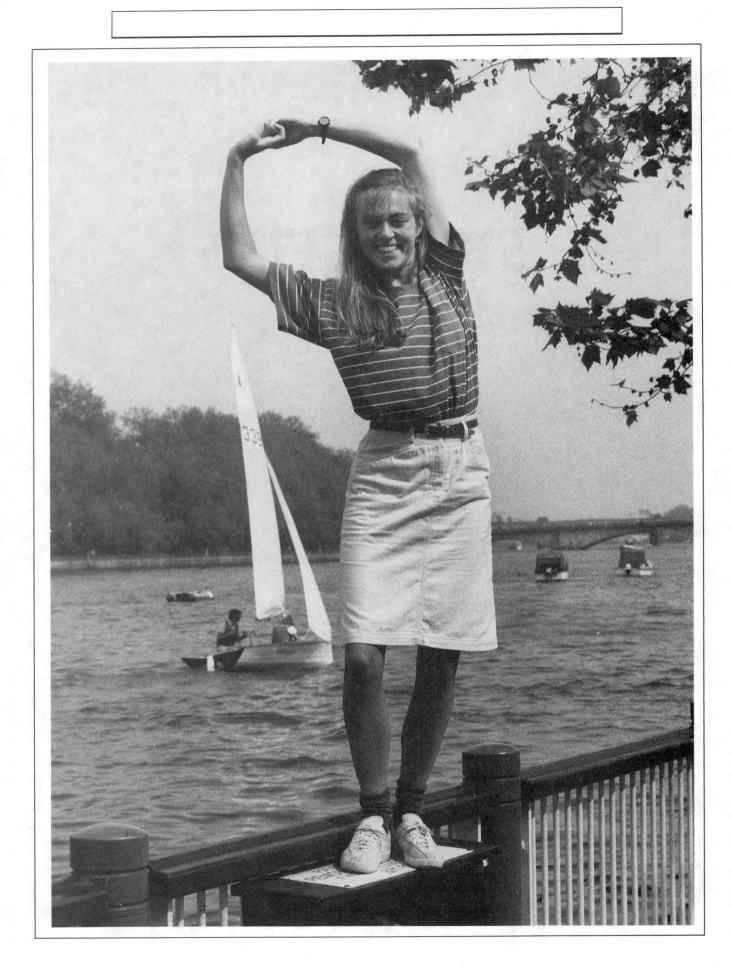

1

Synergetics: A Whole Life Plan

WHAT IS SYNERGETICS?

Synergetics is more than a program of physical exercise, it is a healing and rejuvenation system—a whole life plan. The motions you will learn in the Synergetics system are natural, gentle, and graceful—they allow your mind the serenity to consciously communicate with every part of your body. These motions will help you control your weight, improve your posture, tone your muscles, strengthen your cardiovascular system, and enhance your natural beauty. Synergetics helps to increase your energy and keep everyday stresses from affecting you. The word *Synergetics* describes the way in which the conscious, mind-directed action of every muscle in your body helps every other muscle simultaneously develop its maximum power and ability. Spending 12 minutes practicing these easy motions in the morning, and 12 minutes in the evening, will help regenerate your body, and give you a greater sense of physical and mental well-being.

Synergetics is a total body system that puts no impact or stress on your joints. Every whole-body motion is done standing comfortably upright in one spot, shifting your weight from one foot to the other. The motions are simple and natural. You will use only the built-in strength of your hands and upper body to gently pull or push your torso to its maximum range of motion. Every muscle will work with every other muscle to give you the grace of a ballet dancer and the strength of a weight lifter.

HOW DOES
SYNERGETICS WORK?

Synergetics will relax your mind and body. Rhythmic deep breathing with every motion will enrich your entire system with oxygen, massaging your body internally as well as externally. Your brain and the rest of your body will begin to function better as the circulation of more oxygen, vital body fluids, and body-relaxing substances begins to increase. Stressful mind-chatter will fade as you begin to focus your attention on yourself. Your mind, body, and spirit will come together in a harmony that you may never have experienced before.

Doing Synergetics for 12 minutes before breakfast, and 12 minutes before bedtime (that's less than 2 percent of your day), will help you develop your muscles and your body's natural proportions. In only 24 minutes a day you will be gently flexing every muscle in your body over 700 times a day. In a week you will have flexed every muscle with good resistance almost 5,000 times! You will have a wonderful workout without panting, without sweating, and with no impact on your joints.

The cumulative effect of these motions, and Power Breathing with every flex, stimulates your body's fat burning furnaces, called *mitochondria,* producing the energy needed for muscle contraction—the toning process for every muscle in your body. As your muscle mass increases, your more efficient metabolism will gradually decrease your percentage of excess body fat. The frequency of short Synergetics workouts will effectively increase the rate at which your body burns calories, assisting you in losing weight as your body begins to take on more desirable proportions.

As your circulation improves, you will experience many internal changes. Synergetics stimulates the muscles of your large intestine and colon which in turn makes your body more efficient at digesting food, absorbing nutrients, and eliminating wastes. You may notice a decrease in blood pressure as your increased physical activity increases the efficiency of your circulatory system. Your heart will become stronger as you gently increase your heartbeat for 12 minutes twice a day. You will experience a surge in energy and a lightness in your body. Every day you will feel stronger as you decrease your percentage of fat and increase your muscle mass. You will achieve the balance and agility that you normally see only in trained athletes. You will stand taller without conscious effort. Your body will have a youthful look because of the way you carry yourself. You will feel a sense of well-being—an elation that comes with being proud of yourself and what you are doing.

WILL SYNERGETICS
WORK FOR ME?

By following the program faithfully, you can develop and maintain an athletic and energetic body. The true test will come in a few weeks when you ask yourself: How do I feel? How do I look? Your body and feelings won't lie to you. Your body and your mind will respond to Synergetics because this exercise system closely imitates the motions that your body was built to perform.

In this section we will provide the answers to some of the most common questions people have about Synergetics. Use these answers as a starting point for your own personal philosophy of health. As you begin to learn Synergetics, you will become more conscious of your physical, emotional, and mental processes. Listen carefully to the messages that your body and mind are sending you, follow their instructions, and trust in yourself. If you haven't had a recent medical checkup, get one. It's very important that you know what your present physical condition is so you can set realistic goals and keep yourself in perfect working condition.

IS SYNERGETICS EASY TO LEARN?

You can learn the basic motions in just a few days, by yourself, in front of a mirror. In a very short time the Synergetics motions will become second nature to you. The best way to learn is a little at a time. You will practice the basics until you feel comfortable with them. By this method, you will be able to take the time you need to develop a permanent plan for keeping your body fit. You don't have to rush through the program if you feel like taking more time. Learning a little at a time will allow you to master the proper form for each motion and will let your mind and body learn to do each exercise naturally.

WHAT IS THE IMPORTANCE OF BRINGING YOUR BODY, MIND, AND SPIRIT TOGETHER?

Harmonizing the powers of your body, mind, and spirit is the only way that you can achieve perfect health. For over a thousand years people have practiced Yoga in order to consciously coordinate the body's health with the health of the mind. For generations, the Chinese have practiced Tai Chi Ch'uan in order to bring about a harmony between the body, mind, and spirit. And in recent years this same mind-body-spirit concept—the holistic approach—has attracted many people in search of better health.

Synergetics combines many of the motions of Tai Chi Ch'uan and Yoga to strengthen your body, beautify your face, and bring your conscious mind closer to the natural workings of your body. The Yoga and Tai Chi Ch'uan philosophies of health have now been scientifically proven. *You can't have a healthy body without a healthy mind!* Experiments have shown that the health of the body is directly influenced by what a person thinks and feels.

HOW DOES SYNERGETICS COMPARE WITH TAI CHI CH'UAN?

Tai Chi Ch'uan was originally developed as a martial art (fighting without weapons)—later popularized as purely exercise—while Synergetics was developed strictly as a health system for exercising your body and your mind. Both exercises have much in common, yet there is much that distinguishes the two. In his book *Fundamentals of Tai Chi Ch'uan,* Wen-shan Huang describes the Tai Chi Ch'uan motions by saying:

> They are basically slow, continuous, light, gentle, circular, rhythmic, energetic and graceful movements which are capable of developing an "intrinsic energy," ready to tune up the body, slow down the aging processes, and stretch out the life span of the human body. Each movement also involves the alternate shifting of the body weight from one leg to another and is always synchronized with breathing. Movements are also performed with all parts of the body in unison and harmony to constitute a concerted act of the feet (toes, soles, heels), legs (knees), waist, abdomen, shoulders, neck, head (with eyes watching and ears listening), arms, elbows and hands (palms, fingers). With the spine and waist as sustaining pillar and axis and the feet firmly rooted aground, all other parts of the body are maneuvered, in pairs and fours, simultaneously and rhythmically. . . .

Synergetics embodies these exercise elements in easy flexing/resistance/breathing/posture motions that condition all of your body's parts simultaneously, putting emphasis on flexibility, strength, body alignment, balance, facial flexing, and cardiovascular fitness.

You will learn how to gracefully shift your weight from one foot to the other, as you slowly pull or push your torso into a gentle twist or bend (toning your legs and buttocks as you gain more flexibility and balance). You will learn how to exercise your upper body using the power of your joined hands in either a pulling or pushing position (increasing your functional strength and developing more beautiful upper body contours). You will learn a new method of breathing which will dramatically increase the amount of oxygen you can deliver to your system with every breath (conditioning your cardiovascular system, improving your metabolism, and trimming your waist). You will learn how to develop your muscles so that your body will stand straight and tall without conscious effort. Finally, you will learn flexing motions for your face which will reduce stress, erase wrinkles, and regenerate sagging muscles that cause lines, wrinkles, and double chins.

Wen-shan Huang describes the benefits of Tai Chi Ch'uan by saying:

> It is the combined effect of activated nervous communication, stimulated blood circulation, intensified flowing and draining of the lymphatic fluid and integrated mental relaxation. No wonder it is generally considered as the most successful system of internal and external training, embracing the best principles of modern psychology, physiology, biology, mental hygiene, and dynamics for the promotion of health.

Synergetics simplifies and emphasizes many of the Tai Chi Ch'uan motions and incorporates new motions in a way that produces faster and more dramatic results:

By doing every motion on the balls of your feet, you get the benefits of ballet training for balance and agility, along with additional strength and muscle tone for your legs and buttocks.

By bending or twisting your body to its maximum range with every motion, your muscles become smooth, strong, and Yoga-flexible.

By keeping your head fixed as you move, you are using your spine as your body's axis, which creates more flexing benefits and ability to balance and coordinate your body.

By adding the forceful pulling and pushing of your hands against each other, you get the benefits of a resistance exercise, which is necessary for developing your upper body strength and toning your muscles.

By Power Breathing with every flex, you get the benefits of aerobic dancing. *You increase your heart rate without strain* and trim your waist.

By standing tall as you do the motions, you develop muscles that will hold your body naturally in its most attractive and healthful posture.

By doing facial flexes with every motion, you are releasing stress and recapturing the youthful tone and look of your face.

IS SYNERGETICS LIKE YOGA?

Synergetics is similar to Yoga primarily in its emphasis on proper breathing and stretching, and both exercise disciplines promote relaxation, balance, grace, and flexibility. Yoga focuses on stretching the body from varied positions and practicing the Complete Breath, which is similar to Synergetics Power Breathing. Synergetics also stretches the spine and other parts of the body with every flexing motion, but all of the Synergetics motions are performed standing naturally upright, whereas many Yoga postures are performed sitting or lying on the floor.

Yoga means "union" or "joining together" in Sanskrit—a union of the body, the mind, and the spirit. Although Yoga has been practiced in Eastern cultures for centuries, many people in the West are just now discovering its wonderful ways of keeping their bodies, minds, and spirits in harmony.

WHAT TYPE OF MUSCLE DEVELOPMENT SHOULD I EXPECT?

Gender and body type have a lot to do with the way your body develops. Unless you were, or are a trained athlete, you probably haven't ever developed your physical potential. Your body is unique. You have a different bone structure, a different number of muscle fibers, and a different number of fat cells, all distributed in a unique way in your unique body. As you exercise regularly, the shape of your body will gradually change into its most desirable form. Your body will become more graceful, strong, and shapely. Since every motion stretches your entire body, your muscles will become long, smooth, strong, contoured, and very quick.

CAN I DEVELOP MUSCLE AT ANY AGE WITHOUT HURTING MYSELF?

Yes. There have been recent scientific studies by Priscilla Clarkson, Ph.D. at the University of Massachusetts in Amherst which show that active older people have the same ability to safely increase their strength as college students, although it may take a little longer. In an article, "Sore Muscles," William Stockton, a *New York Times* writer, reports on her work:

> . . . What scientists have found is that when we exercise a muscle and put some unaccustomed stress on it, the muscle is damaged slightly. Some of the muscle fibers become torn or broken and proteins and enzymes "leak" out of the muscle cells.

> But the significant discovery was that after the muscle repairs itself, it is more resistant to injury than before.

> In fact, just a single exercise session can induce this adaptation, and the effects can last for several weeks. And as they have narrowed their focus on this training effect, Clarkson and her colleagues have found that a minimal workout that puts just enough stress on a muscle can result in a muscle a few days later that can perform a strenuous exercise without damage. Such a feat would have been impossible without serious damage before the training session.

> The trick is to put just enough stress on the muscle, but not too much. Overdo it and the damage can become so substantial that days or weeks can be lost while the muscle recovers. . . .

> . . . begin slowly, pushing your muscles slightly the first day and continuing to up the ante day by day. In the long run, the results will be greater, Clarkson contends. . . .

> The researchers have also extended the research to older people, comparing their muscles with those of college students.

> They have found that the older people—average age 67.4 years and very active—have the same ability to adapt to muscle damage and that the muscle repair process is equally effective as in the young people. Subsequent research has shown, however, that strength may return more slowly in the older people.

Regardless of your age, with few exceptions, you can gradually and safely increase your muscle development and functional power by simply following the Synergetics philosophy of using your own, built-in body strength to exercise yourself.

HOW QUICKLY WILL I SEE RESULTS?

Your progress will depend on your present condition and your commitment to the twice daily Synergetics program. The program recommends that you work out twice a day: 12 minutes in the morning and 12 minutes in the evening. This is the ideal schedule for optimum results. However, there may be times when you can only work out once a day, or just a few times a week. Work out with Synergetics whenever you can and wherever you can, always shooting for the ideal, because a little bit is better than nothing at all.

You will probably *feel* the results first: more energy, less stress, better elimination, a feeling of strength and quickness, and clearer thinking. Some people see physical results in just a few days, or within a week or so. Much depends on your age and present physical condition. Some bodies may respond more quickly to the exercises because of previous athletic training. Usually, your measurements will begin to change, first with inches lost in different parts of your body. If you are overweight, you might begin to experience a gradual weight loss as your muscles develop (keep in mind that muscle weighs more than fat—so don't go by the scales alone). You will notice more muscle definition as well as a more youthful look to your face. Friends and family seem to notice the changes first, even without knowing that you are working on making changes.

WHAT ABOUT DIETING?

Most health experts agree that drastic dieting rarely works for losing weight, and often upsets your metabolism. However, monitoring the amount of food you eat, and the quality of the food you eat, is essential. Most of us don't grow our own food, but we all have a choice of how we feed our bodies. We can eat out of flashy plastic packages with photographs on the label showing what the food used to look like (food that is now loaded with sugar, refined flour, and chemicals), or we can nourish our irreplaceable, one and only bodies with fresh, natural, unprocessed foods.

You must learn how to eat naturally. Your body evolved by eating "live" foods— foods containing live enzymes which are essential for absorbing whatever nutrition the food contains. Your body is genetically programmed to process high-fiber, untainted foods like fresh fruits and vegetables, whole grain breads, a little fresh meat, and a lot of pure water. Anything less begins to prematurely age your organs and your entire body.

Fat will begin to form in excessive amounts on your body from over-caloried manufactured foods; your blood sugar level will begin to go up and down like a yo-yo from the excessive shocks of heavily sugared products; your digestive tract and colon will spasm and get inflamed from a thick, pasty coating of refined flour products; your blood will begin to fill with a waxy substance called cholesterol—from eating too many animal/dairy products—which slowly but surely builds up on the walls of your veins and arteries, closing off your lifeline of blood until you could have a heart attack and die.

Sounds pretty grim, doesn't it? Well it is. The populations of three dozen foreign countries have a greater life expectancy than we do. In this country we spend almost as much on medical care every year as we do on food.

Go to your kitchen right now. Take all of the packaged and canned foods you have and line them up on your counter. Now read the labels one by one—marking a big *X* (a symbol for poison) on the ones that are full of sugar (and its derivatives) and refined flour. Do the same for any foods that have a list of chemicals on the label that you know nothing about. Food processors had to be *forced* to quit putting red dye and sulphites in their foods, even though they are known to kill humans. Can you trust them now? If you have enough food without an *X* left for supper, then you are eating better than the average person in this country.

Go to your bookstore or health food store and get some current books on nutrition and whole foods cooking. Study them. Become an expert on how to keep yourself and your family healthy and alive. You must know for yourself, and have a clear understanding of what's good for you and what isn't, before you can become determined and committed to do something positive about the deadly drift of our country toward nutritional collapse.

So don't think *diet*. Think *nutrition*. Counting and measuring calories can throw your body into a physiological tizzy. Eating the most nutritious, natural food you can find is the simple way to give your body the health, energy, and beauty it deserves.

CAN I LOSE WEIGHT WITH SYNERGETICS?

Yes. The amount of weight you lose will depend on your specific body type, your present physical condition, as well as the timing, frequency, duration, and intensity of your workouts. According to one study, the best time of the day to exercise is early in the morning. Professor Anthony Wilcox, in a 1986 study at Kansas State University, found that you burn the same amount of calories no matter what time of day you exercise, but if you exercise early in the morning you will burn mostly fat calories. And if you exercise in the afternoon, you will burn mostly carbohydrate calories. You can trim down a lot faster by burning fat. The recommended time for your first Synergetics workout is right before breakfast.

According to a study reported in *The Rejuvenation Strategy* by René Cailliet, M.D. and Leonard Gross, athletes were able to increase their metabolic rate (calorie burning rate) by as much as 25 percent for 24 hours with a brisk morning workout. By permanently increasing your metabolic rate (the process by which you turn food into energy and living tissue), you can gradually lose excess pounds until you reach a plateau of perfect weight for your body type.

The recommended time for your last workout of the day is right before bedtime. Instead of going to bed with a "sleepy" metabolic rate, you can again tune your body to burn additional calories all night long while you sleep with a series of gentle Synergetics motions. Not only does this workout wake up your metabolism, but it also helps trigger a natural, body-relaxing, stress-relieving, narcoticlike brain compound called *endorphins*.

How many times a day you work out, when you work out, how long you work out, how hard you work out, and what you eat are going to determine how much and how fast you lose excess body fat. Be patient with yourself, take your time, lose weight gradually, and enjoy your new lifestyle as you make your permanent changes.

CAN I GET RID OF CELLULITE?

If you can get rid of body fat, you can get rid of cellulite, because that's what cellulite is: excess fat that has built up in certain spots on your body and which has broken through some of the natural netting of your tissue just under your skin, causing dimpling.

For decades, people desperate to get rid of cellulite dimpling have subjected themselves to *spot exercising, spot surgery,* and now *spot liposuction* with not-so-satisfactory results. First of all, spot exercising doesn't selectively get rid of cellulite in one particular spot because the body uses its fat from all of its parts for energy—not from one specific area. Second, and most important, removing fat cells from your body surgically or by liposuction is an unhealthy shock to your body, which is genetically programmed to function with a certain number of fat cells. Recently there have been reports that the body will begin to create new fat cells to replace the ones that were torn from the body by unnatural means, so you would be right back where you started after risking your health with potentially dangerous and unnecessary surgery.

If you really are serious about getting rid of your cellulite, then begin eating a diet of fresh vegetables, fruit, rice, potatoes, grains, beans, etc., and a very small amount of animal and dairy products, or anything that contains sugar or refined flour. Think carefully about the foods you've been eating and consult with your physician to get advice on better eating habits. Add a daily program of Synergetics to your new eating habits, and in a few months you will have dramatically changed your body's dimensions and reduced the dimples to nothing but smooth, firm flesh.

WILL SYNERGETICS GIVE ME CARDIOVASCULAR CONDITIONING?

Synergetics is a safe, no-impact alternative to the "go for the burn" aerobic exercises of the seventies and eighties. The problem with strenuous aerobic exercises like high-speed calisthenics, jazz dancing, and jogging, is that they keep the heart in good shape but they often destroy the body's bone structure. And many of the so-called soft aerobic programs aren't soft at all; they are designed primarily for young bodies with a great deal of athletic ability and endurance.

With Synergetics, the no-impact action of shifting your weight from the ball of one foot to the other, with your knees slightly bent, gently increases your blood circulation in your lower extremities. It's a stalking type of motion that gives your legs more of a flex. The steady force that you exert on your hands as you slowly pull or push your body to its maximum twist or bend creates a muscle-pumping action that pulls blood through your upper body. The deep breathing technique increases the volume of oxygen that you are able to take in with every inhale and decreases the amount of spent air that you leave in your body on every exhale. The combined leg and upper body action, coupled with steady force on your hands along with deep breathing, increases your heart rate in a safe and gradual way.

You can increase the tempo of your repetitions and increase the force that you use on your hands to increase your heart rate. Since Synergetics uses the actions and the strengths of your own body (and not a machine), and since you are not required to run, jump, wiggle, swing, or kick, there is no excess impact on your joints or danger of hurting yourself.

The word *aerobic* is defined as any activity in the presence of oxygen. Synergetics can give you the degree of aerobic activity you desire. Synergetics can be used as a gentle, right-before-going-to-bed, stress-relieving, metabolism-priming ritual, or as a replacement for jogging, aerobic dancing, or high-speed calisthenics. You can pace yourself, using your built-in instincts to tell you how much action your body needs at any given time, and bring your heart rate up to the level you would get if you briskly jogged a mile or two. Since you are purposely forcing added oxygen into your lungs rather than being forced to gasp for it (as in strenuous aerobics), there is no danger of straining your heart from lack of oxygen. If you are deep breathing properly, you should be able to carry on a normal conversation right after you have ended your workout without being short of breath.

In two moderate, 12-minute Synergetics workouts a day you will flex your body more than 700 times, shift your weight almost 700 times, and supercharge your body with almost 400 deep breaths (2 seconds per flex, or 4 seconds for a complete back and forth motion). If you choose to work at the *Breezing Tempo,* you can double the above figures and build your endurance dramatically. It stands to reason that fourteen moderate, 12-minute workouts a week will give you a more efficiently conditioned cardiovascular system than three strenuous 20- or 30-minute workouts a week. The Synergetics program is also safer. Your body works best if it has more frequent, shorter sessions of concentrated physical activity.

THE NUMBERS GAME

The old "heart-rated" exercise schools decree that you have to exercise for 20 to 30 minutes, three times a week, at a heart rate of 180 heartbeats minus your age, or 220 heartbeats minus your age multiplied by .60, .70, or .80 (depending on your present physical condition). This means that if you are forty years old you have to maintain a heart rate (beats per minute) of 140 (180 minus 40) for a minimum of 20 minutes to get cardiovascular benefit. This regimen may be medically sound for your heart, but what good is an exercise program if you aren't physically able or willing to do it? Are you willing to voluntarily make three appointments a week to work your body to the point of exhaustion and risk permanently injuring your joints? Think about it.

What should your blood pressure be for your age? 120/80? 115/75? 106/66? What should your resting pulse rate be? 60? 70? 80? 90? What should your target heart rate be (the number of beats per minute to which you should try to elevate your heart rate for cardiovascular conditioning)? 120? 130? 140? These questions can't be answered unless you have a complete physical examination by a specialist in this particular field. You can measure your own heart rate (beats per minute) by placing your first three fingers on the artery on the side of your neck just under your jawbone, counting the beats for 15 seconds, then multiplying by 4.

Be wary of trying to get your heart rate up to the "recommended heart rate numbers" unless you are sure you are in excellent physical shape. Do you have a latent heart defect? Or maybe a heavy buildup of cholesterol in your blood vessels? Why not get a thorough medical checkup and be sure of your present physical condition? Show Synergetics to your physician and follow his or her advice. Work against your own standard, not some statistical table. If your doctor tells you that your blood pressure is too high, or that your cholesterol count is too high, or that you are overweight for your body type and height, and that you have too high a fat to muscle ratio, then take notes, make goals, and do something about your condition.

The following article, written by Nanci Hellmich, cites a study which shows that shorter workouts (12 minutes) are giving people good aerobic results. From *USA Today*, June 1988:

Aerobics fans can get good results with shorter workouts, a new study indicates.

Working out as little as 12 minutes, three times a week improves your cardiovascular fitness, researchers found. Standing recommendations: 20–30 minutes, three times a week.

"People may be putting themselves through needlessly long workouts," says Dr. James Rippe, a cardiologist and director of the exercise physiology laboratory at the University of Massachusetts Medical School. . . .

In the past it has been cast in stone that to derive aerobic benefit you must exercise 20 to 30 minutes with aerobics.

Researchers had twenty-three women in average shape ride a computerized stationary bike for 12 minutes three times a week. They increased cardiovascular fitness by 5 percent in two weeks, 11 percent in twelve weeks.

The study doesn't mean you don't derive additional benefits from 30-minute workouts, Dr. Rippe says, but 12 minutes accomplishes what are viewed as excellent results.

If just 12 minutes, three times a week, of bike riding is helpful, think how you would look and feel if you integrated two, 12-minute Synergetics workouts into your everyday schedule. Even though you could probably survive on just three meals a week and three nights of sleep a week, you will obviously feel much better when you eat and sleep on a daily schedule. Your body is designed to function better if it has daily exercise, too. Cleaning your house, seasonal gardening, weekend sports, and three workouts a week are not enough. Your body needs concentrated physical activity several times a day—much, much more than the average person gets these days.

Synergetics is another name for the natural motions of your body, and these motions can condition your cardiovascular system naturally—allowing your body to use all of its muscles in a single, coordinated motion in an upright position which helps circulate your blood more efficiently. You will feel the results of your workouts and see positive physical results as well. Make a point of getting regular checkups from your doctor and let him keep track of the blood pressure and pulse numbers for you.

For optimum cardiovascular conditioning, always do a series of the Leg Synergetics in conjunction with the Rainbows at a brisk tempo.

WHY SHOULDN'T I SWEAT?

Sweating is not necessary for fitness. Sweat has always been associated with fitness, because most types of exercise cause us to sweat by overheating our bodies. A few beads of perspiration won't hurt, but the "sweat and burn" that many exercise programs promote, robs your body of fluid which is filled with essential minerals, salts, and electrolytes—all vital to your health and energy. Remember when you got dizzy or sick to your stomach after a strenuous workout? Your body was telling you to leave its fluid level alone and to quit overheating it! How many times have you heard someone say: "I ran five miles today and lost three pounds!" They did lose three pounds—three pounds in body fluid that must be replaced or they could become dehydrated and ill. In a day or two their weight is right back where it started. Their body was unnecessarily abused.

If you love the feel of sweat smarting in your eyes as the beads trickle down your face and drip off your nose, and if dark patches of wetness on your clothes are fitness symbols to you, then go for the burn. But, if you want to conserve your energy, your clothes, your precious time, and your one-and-only body, forget the sweat.

IS SYNERGETICS SAFE?

If you have an injury or condition that could be aggravated by even a gentle workout routine, consult your physician before beginning any new exercise program.

Synergetics can help with lower back problems by relieving stress, improving spine alignment, repositioning spinal disks, and strengthening abdominal muscles (which helps take the stress off the lower back). The motions are excellent, in many cases, for injury rehabilitation, since they can be done very gently to safely build up damaged parts of the body. It is important to ask yourself, What are you trying to accomplish with your exercise program? Are you training for the Boston Marathon? Getting ready for another pro football season with the New York Giants? Or, trying to get fit so that you can enjoy an active lifestyle? If you just want to stay fit, then play it safe and avoid overdoing your exercises.

YOUR COMMON SENSE DEGREE

Many of the questions that we depend on others to answer for us, we can answer for ourselves. We are all born with a degree even more valuable than an M.D. or a Ph.D. It's our C.S.D. (Common Sense Degree). Even though we all have it, we sometimes ignore it, forgetting that common sense can give us the real answers. We have access to a built-in computer that has conceived and built rocket ships and radio telescopes, yet we rarely use more than a small fraction of it to manage our own daily lives. We tend to surrender ourselves to other people who can't possibly know how our bodies are feeling inside. Sometimes we search out people to tell us what we *want* to hear, rather than what we *need* to hear. It's a lifelong quest, but the rewards for using more of our C.S.D. are worth it.

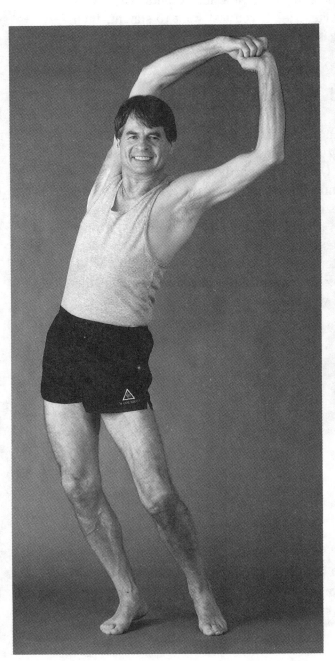

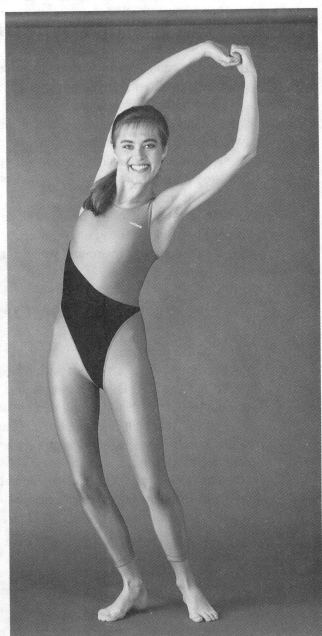

2

Synergetics Tips

CLIMBING A RAINBOW

Forming a new exercise habit can be quite a challenge—like trying to find that legendary pot of gold at the end of a rainbow. With Synergetics you may be doing the opposite—trying to get rid of another kind of "pot" that is easily located by just looking in your mirror. Even though you are investing only 24 minutes a day (12 minutes before breakfast, and 12 minutes before bedtime), your old habits may come back to haunt you and make you forget to exercise. Two workouts a day is ideal, but don't feel guilty or get discouraged if your routine isn't as consistent as it should be—it will come in time.

- When you first begin Synergetics, you may get the same feeling you had when you tried to pat your head and rub your stomach at the same time. This feeling will go away in several days. You can help your body get used to the motions by taking them one at a time, and practicing each one until the motions become second nature.

- Even though the motions are done slowly and easily, you are going to feel your muscles beginning to stretch and strengthen almost immediately. You will feel every muscle in your body becoming alive—fatty tissue breaking down and muscles beginning to regenerate themselves. For relaxation you can give yourself a light self-massage right after your workout to aid this new level of blood circulation and muscle regeneration in your body.

- You may find that you never sweat while you are doing Synergetics. Unless you are out in the hot sun, or in a very warm room, or doing Synergetics at a fast tempo, you may find that you can do your workout even after you have had your bath, or are fully dressed, without perspiring.

- You may feel a little lightheaded at first, because you are breathing more deeply than you normally do. This is natural, and will not last as you learn to completely exhale the spent air (mostly carbon dioxide). Be sure your breaths are deep and slow, rather than shallow and fast. Always breathe with a powerful, rhythmic tempo. If a feeling of dizziness persists, be sure to see your doctor.

- You will never be bored while you are doing Synergetics, because you can occupy your mind with other things while you are working out. You can enjoy watching the changes in your body in your mirror, watching TV (after you have mastered the motions), moving to your favorite music, or just letting your mind float in meditation.

- Make Synergetics part of your daily life, and a natural part of your body's functions, like stretching and yawning. As soon as your body accepts this twice daily relaxing interlude, Synergetics will become a necessary part of your life like eating and sleeping. Your body will crave (and welcome) your twice daily workouts.

BEFORE YOU BEGIN

Read and follow the step by step instructions carefully. The benefits of Synergetics are directly proportional to how closely you can duplicate the motions. There are many subtle, but important differences between Synergetics motions and other exercises that you may have learned in the past.

- Don't try to learn every exercise on the first day. Master one Synergetics motion at a time and then go on to the next one. Although it is important to develop a full program of Synergetics motions, one exercise done correctly for 12 minutes twice a day can condition every muscle in your body.

- Exercise every day, twice a day, preferably right when you get up in the morning and right before you go to bed. These times were chosen for physiological reasons as well as for convenience. A minimum of 12 solid minutes of Synergetics per workout is recommended for the cardiovascular effect as well as for strength and endurance training.

- Do any number of Synergetics, anytime, anywhere. One minute of Synergetics will help relieve stress and anxiety, 3 minutes will help curb your appetite and increase your energy, and 12 minutes twice a day will keep you fit. Take every opportunity to give your body a Synergetics break during the day—in the kitchen, in the office, in the restroom—wherever you are.

- Learn Synergetics in front of a mirror. All of the photographs in this book reflect your mirror image (as if you were looking into the mirror at yourself). Coach yourself in front of the mirror to be sure you are standing tall with your chin tucked in and with your head always fixed in one position.

- Dress however you like. You can exercise in workout clothes, business clothes, or with no clothes at all. Since you don't have to sweat or get down on the floor to do Synergetics you have more options on how you dress.

- Weigh yourself morning and evening—right before you exercise. As you step onto the scale, concentrate on the weight you want to be, not the weight you want to lose. This is an effective method for giving your unconscious mind positive direction. If you hate your present weight, or hate your fat, or hate your body, your unconscious will fight to protect it just the way it is. But if you let go of the negative feelings and concentrate with positive feelings on how you want to look, your unconscious will help you lose the pounds. When the scale registers your present weight, again register a positive thought of what you want to weigh. Avoid any feeling of impatience or frustration with yourself.

- Sip a small glass of fruit juice while you are exercising. Juice will prime your body (especially in the morning) so you won't get weak or dizzy from low blood sugar.

- Train your mind to concentrate on every motion in your 12-minute workout. Concentrating on every move will keep your body from getting lazy, and will help focus your mind on making positive changes. Try to get the same feeling of physical and mental readiness that you would feel just before you jump off of a diving board or as you answer the ring of your telephone.

- Exercise with your favorite music. Music is fun to move with. The Synergetics motions are done just like a dance step, shifting your weight from one foot to the other and moving your body in a smooth rhythm to the beat of the music. If the music is too fast to keep up with every beat, do your motions with a half-time rhythm. Music is a great motivator to get your body moving!

- Doing Synergetics while watching your favorite TV programs can be a great way to get in shape. You're not taking out additional time from your day, and you can get a good workout by just doing your exercises during the commercials.

- Or you can exercise in total silence, letting your mind relax and float. This meditation in motion can be a great energizer and rejuvenator.

- Relax. Your Synergetics workout is meant to be a mind-calming, body-relaxing event. Forget the frantic exercises of the past, and experience a new form of relaxation in motion.

- Become graceful, making every motion like a ballet step. The 1-2-3, step by step instructions are meant to be blended into one continuous, flowing, back and forth motion.

- Don't give up! Synergetics is your first best step to better health. Learn and master the motions and do them twice a day, even if your untrained body wants to give up.

- Smile! This is the most important Synergetics exercise of all! A smile or a laugh will instantly flood your body with more stress-relieving substances than two weeks in the Bahamas. Try a really broad smile right this instant. Feel the difference? Smiling for 12 minutes, twice a day will make a wonderful difference in your life.

MIND POWER

Your thoughts will become your feelings, your feelings will become your actions, your actions will become your habits, and your habits will become part of your every-day routine. So what you think and feel is very important. What do you want to be? Until you have a clear mental picture of how you want to feel, how you want to look, and who you want to be, you will have a hard time becoming your best self.

Emile Coué, the father of autosuggestion, and author of the saying, "Day by day, in every way, I'm getting better and better," said, "Always think of what you have to do as easy and it will become so." Most of your great achievements begin in your mind, so you must first consciously decide what you want to accomplish, and then think of it as easy so you will not be afraid to go for it.

Mentally image what you want your body to become, and how you want it to feel, and work through the Synergetics training program at your own pace, until you reach the level of physical and mental fitness that satisfies you. Then establish a maintenance program that fits your mind's and body's needs.

Imaging is mentally and emotionally "picturing" the physical and mental changes that you want to make in yourself, and then focusing on these images for a few minutes during your day. *Imaging gives you the power to make the physical and mental changes that will enrich your life.*

- First, you must figure out what you want to look like and feel like. Close your eyes. Sketch a mental picture of the way you would like to look and feel. Highlight your best features and most positive feelings. Imagine a terrific, new, energetic you. Got a clear picture? Now, how do you want to feel? Relaxed? Happy? Serene? Secure? Strong? Attractive? Confident?

- Now, close your eyes again and think about the real reason why you want to get in good shape by asking yourself these questions: Do you want to get in shape in order to be attractive? To compete in athletics? To avoid surgery? To keep from looking old? To save your life? To look better in clothes? To get along better with people? To feel better? To compete in business? To have more energy? To have a longer health span? To dance better? To be proud of yourself? To be strong enough to care for the ones you love? To get along better with yourself?

- Open your eyes. Now make some notes for yourself. Describe how you want to feel, what changes you want to make, and what outcomes—what results you want for yourself. Then, make a list of your reasons for getting into shape. Remember, be honest and realistic with yourself.

• Twice a day, right before your Synergetics workout, study the outcomes and changes you have listed for yourself. Then, as you do your 12-minute workout, concentrate on one of the most important changes you listed and think about why you want to make that change. Mentally work on one change at a time. Eventually, they will all come true. Add new ideas to your list as they come to you.

Using the power of your mind to help you become what you want to be is the secret to forming a Synergetics lifestyle. And this same power will motivate you to whisper to yourself twenty times every morning before you get out of bed, and twenty times every night just before you go to sleep, "Day by day, in every way, I'm getting better and better." (More on Autosuggestion in Chapter 11.)

LET'S BEGIN!

The next few weeks could be the most exciting and fulfilling time of your life. You will be concentrating on, and working with, the most important person in the world—you! Begin to think of yourself as an ever-improving person with built-in powers that are just waiting to be released through positive physical and mental actions.

You will notice that the exercise sequences of the daily programs are varied to keep your body in a constant state of surprise. If your body ever gets into a "ho-hum, this is too easy" state, then you might as well stop your workout, climb into bed, and take a nap.

Every day your body will gain more strength with which to exercise itself. Be conscious of your increased strength, and bear down a little more with the pulling and pushing of your hands so that your body is always challenged. When the motions become too easy from lack of hand resistance, you will not get the full benefits from your workout. So be sure to keep a steady, strong force on your hands, and if your body asks for it, pick up the tempo a little.

After you have carefully learned all of the basic Synergetics motions, the daily programs should take approximately 12 minutes from start to finish. Some days your workout may take a little longer, depending on how quickly you pick up on the new motions. Be sure to complete the daily and weekly programs before you settle on one or more routines for your ongoing Synergetics program. If you skip any of the step by step training programs, then you will miss out on some important lessons that will give you the changes you want for your body.

SAFETY CHECKS

You are the world's foremost authority on your body, so listen to what your body tells you and follow its instructions.

Let's review a few safety tips for you to keep in mind as you build or rebuild your body:

- If you get dizzy, shaky, or weak, immediately relax with your hands on your hips, or sit down on the floor for a moment. Feeling weak is not normal. Be sure that you have enough fruit juice or energy food in your body before beginning your workout. And inhale slowly and exhale completely.

- If you feel a muscle begin to pull or spasm, stop immediately and gently massage the area until it relaxes. Then, very slowly try some more motions. If the muscle starts to pull again, omit that particular motion until you feel your muscle is ready to continue exercising. The problem may be due to lack of oxygen to that part of your body, which allows acid byproducts of metabolism to build up in your muscle fiber, causing burning sensations and cramps. Breathe deeply and slowly with every motion to assure that your body receives its optimum amount of oxygen. Don't rush. Build your endurance slowly. Contrary to old-fashioned exercise myths, you don't want to burn!

- If you feel your joints getting sore, you may be jerking, snapping, swinging your body, locking your knees, or collapsing on your hips, which can compress your spine and joints. As you sway or twist, use your good judgment. Be gentle as you pull or push your body to its maximum extension.

If you become worried about a persistent, unpleasant pain or health problem, see your doctor immediately!

BRAINSTORMS AND ENERGY BURSTS

How many times have you wished you had taken the time to write down a great idea—an idea that is now long forgotten? It happens all the time. It might be the solution to a big problem, or an idea for an invention, a poem, a song, or something you want to say to someone, or something you want to remember. The thought flashes through your mind like a comet, and like a comet, quickly disappears into the vastness of your mental universe never to return. Synergetics has a way of releasing these creative flashes. Now, you can store up these brainstorms and make them into realities. Use these semiblank pages as a workbook for your great ideas. Use your book as a sort of mental "comet catcher."

There are progress charts printed on these pages so you can record your chosen changes. You might want to fill this chart out now, before you start, so you will have a record of how you're doing with the goals you choose for yourself.

_____

_____

_____

_____

_____

_____

_____

YOUR PERSONAL PROGRESS RECORD

DATE	WEIGHT	WAIST	HIPS	THIGHS	CHEST	STRENGTH (1–10)
____	_____	_____	____	_____	_____	_____

COORDINATION (1–10)	ENERGY (1–10)	RELAXED (1–10)	SLEEP (1–10)
_____	_____	_____	_____

ELIMINATION (1–10)	EATING HABITS (1–10)	FACE (1–10)	OVERALL APPEARANCE (1–10)
_____	_____	_____	_____

OVERALL FEELINGS (1–10)   NOTE: Score 1 as low and 10 as high.

_____

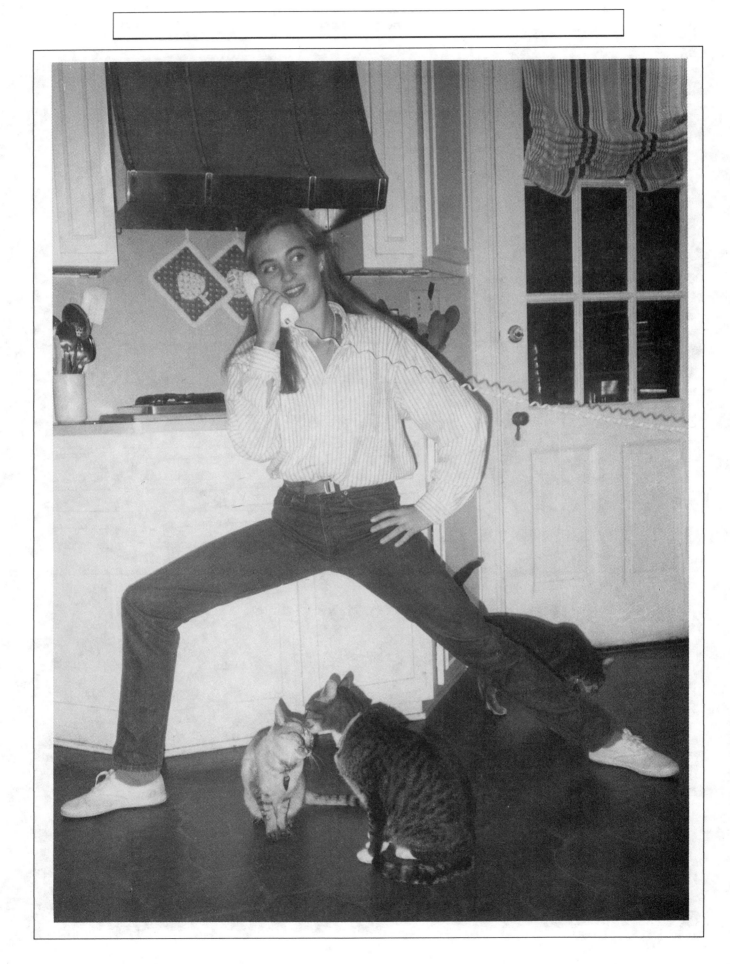

3

Learning
the Basics

Learning how to do Synergetics is like learning a new way to dance. Each dance style, whether it be dancing to a waltz, rock and roll, or the fandango has certain basic moves that are repeated over and over again. After you learn the basic steps, you add variations to make the dance more challenging and fun, just as you add variations to Synergetics to make the exercise more challenging and fun.

Like dancing, Synergetics has rhythm—a tempo—sometimes very slow, and sometimes more lively depending on your mood and energy at the time. And, again like dancing, the motions were created to soothe your body and mind, allowing more positive energy to flow into you, forcing stress and depression to move out and away.

Learning Synergetics can be very easy if you relax your body and open your mind to new possibilities of motion. At first you may feel that you are asking your body to make too many moves simultaneously, even though they are all natural, logical, balanced, and coordinated motions. Make learning the basics a happy experience for yourself. Laugh and chase away frustration when your body becomes a little confused. Remind yourself that Synergetics is a new experience, and your body needs a little time to get used to its unique motions. Then smile smugly in the mirror as you begin to take control of your own body. After you have learned the basic motions, you will begin your 14-day training program, learning Basic and Extended Rainbows, the core exercises of Synergetics.

First, you will learn how to use your body as your own complete "exercise machine." To make Synergetics work, your body must work as a synergetic unit—every muscle helping every other muscle develop itself—every motion flexing every muscle in your body simultaneously—and every motion, every flex becoming grace-ful, balanced, and coordinated. To become athletic and graceful as a ballet dancer, you must practice certain basic moves and postures over and over again so that you build the right habits from the very beginning. Just like your body, these exercises are unique, and must be done correctly so that you can get the most good out of every motion.

Stand in front of your mirror and practice the basic elements until they feel natural to you. All instruction photographs are your mirror image. So, the image you see in the mirror is the same position of the image you will see in this book. Relax. Don't hurry. Don't worry. This is the beginning of a life full of health, energy, and happiness for you!

LOWER BODY MOTION

Foot position, knee flex, hip action, and weight shift. The position of your feet, how you flex your knees, how you move your hips, and the way you shift your weight from one foot to the other will determine the grace and balance of your motions, and how much leg strength and muscle tone you will get from doing Synergetics.

- Your heels should be spaced about 6″ apart with your toes turned out at an angle (the opposite of pigeon-toed). This position will help keep you from losing your balance by rolling over on the side of your foot and you will avoid putting strain on your knee joints as you shift your weight from one foot to the other.

- Your knees should be kept slightly bent (flexed) at all times to keep your body balanced without bobbing up and down, and also to keep you from impacting your body weight on your spine, hip joints, knee joints, and ankle joints. By keeping your knees bent, you will develop strength and leg contour more quickly.

- Your hips must naturally follow the direction of your hands for the best body flex and balance. All but one Synergetics exercise requires that your hips follow your hands into a gentle but tight twist. Imagine you are standing in a small barrel up to your waist and that you don't want to touch the sides as you twist. Only one exercise requires the hip sway (instead of a twist) which gives your spine a different flexing motion.

- All of your weight must be transferred to the ball of one foot, with the other foot barely touching the floor for balance. You should be able to actually lift your nonweight-bearing foot off of the floor if you have shifted your weight properly.

- Practice shifting your weight back and forth until you feel comfortable with the motion. Shift your weight gracefully and rhythmically—two slow counts to the right—two slow counts to the left.

Let's practice the **Weight Shift:**

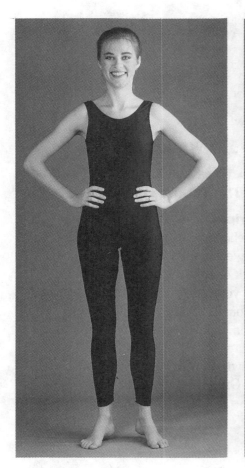 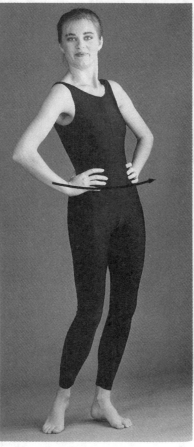 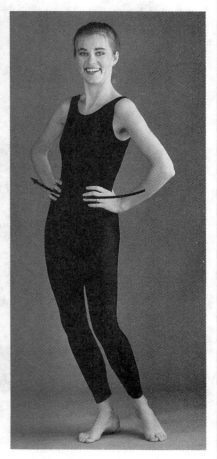

1

Stand with your weight evenly distributed on the balls of both feet. Space your heels about 6" apart with your feet angled out. Bend your knees slightly so that your weight is mostly on the balls of your feet. Tuck your hips under. **Don't stand swaybacked.** If you have difficulty balancing on the balls of your feet, then put some of your weight on your heels until you feel comfortable the other way.

2

Shift your weight to your right foot, keeping your knees slightly bent, and take all of your weight off of your left foot. (To be sure that you've shifted your weight completely, try lifting your left foot a couple of inches off of the floor.) Allow your hips to turn naturally toward the direction you are shifting your weight.

3

Shift your weight to your left foot, keeping your knees slightly bent, and take all of your weight off of your right foot. (To be sure you've shifted your weight completely, try lifting your right foot a couple of inches off of the floor.) Allow your hips to turn naturally toward the direction you are shifting your weight.

THE GRIPS

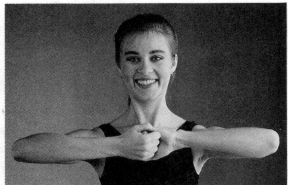

The Finger Hook

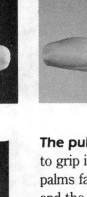

The Thumb Grip

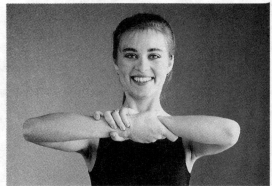

The Wrist Grip

The pull grip. The most effective way to grip is to hook your fingers with your palms facing each other (The Finger Hook) and the back of either your right or left hand facing your body. But if your fingernails are long enough that they dig into your fingers when you pull, grasp your thumbs with your fingers (The Thumb Grip), or grasp your wrists with your fingers (The Wrist Grip). Use the grip that is most comfortable for you.

The push position. Place the tips of your fingers and thumbs together and push through every Synergetics motion with a constant force—pushing with one hand, and resisting with the other.

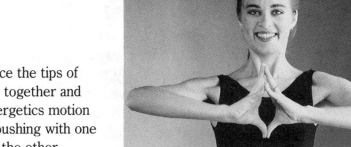

The Fingertip Push

Head and shoulder position. *Always* keep your face straight ahead. *Never* turn or duck your head as you do Synergetics. Only push or pull your body as far as you can without ducking or turning your head away from its original position. Also be careful not to hunch your shoulders up around your ears as you exercise. Go through the motions with your shoulders relaxed, rolled back and down. Notice the muscles in the side of your neck flexing—this is what you want. Keep your head up and your chin tucked in.

Practice this back-and-forth motion as many times as necessary until you get the hang of it.

UPPER BODY MOTION

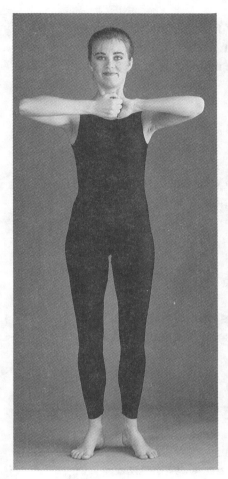

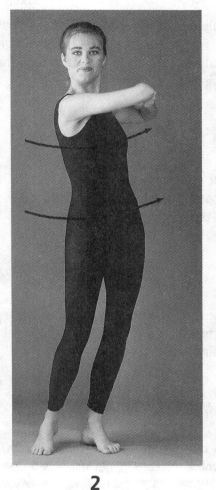

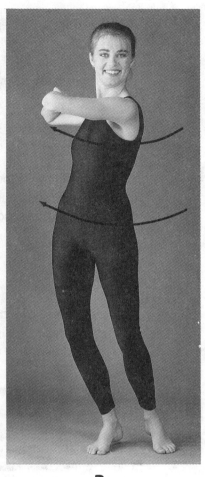

1

Stand as instructed in the Lower Body Motion section. Facing forward, hook your fingers in the pull grip just under your chin, elbows at shoulder height, and relax your shoulders. Hold your head high with your chin in.

2

Keep your face looking straight into your mirror as you slowly pull your hands around to your right as far as you can. Shift all of your weight to the ball of your right foot, gently pulling your body into a right twist. Allow your hips to follow naturally. Don't turn your head or look out of the corners of your eyes! Keep your head full-face to the mirror. Pull with constant force with your right hand and resist with constant force with your left hand.

3

Now, without moving your head one tiny bit, slowly pull your hands back to your left. Shift all of your weight to the ball of your left foot, gently pulling your body into a left twist. Pull with constant force with your left hand and resist with constant force with your right hand. Be sure you watch yourself in a mirror so that you don't turn your head away and look out of the corners of your eyes. You will lose most of the flexing benefits of Synergetics if you do.

BREATHING

For now, practice deeply and slowly inhaling through your nose all the way across the motion, as you pull your hands (and body) to your right. Exhale completely and slowly from your relaxed open mouth all the way across the motion, as you pull your hands (your body following) back to your left.

TEMPO

The Basic Tempo is four seconds, a smooth, slow motion to your right (counting one thousand one, one thousand two), and a smooth, slow motion back to your left (counting one thousand three, one thousand four).

SMILE!

This motion can't be mentioned often enough. Your smile is central to the health of your entire being. It signals all of your 200 trillion body cells that you feel good about yourself and that they should feel good too. And they will!

ON YOUR MARK, GET SET—

Now you are ready to begin your 14-day training program—the Rainbow Series. These exercises are called Rainbows because they exercise your entire muscle structure by moving your interlocked hands in a rainbowlike arc through multiple positions around your body.

During this same two week period you will practice and learn Power Breathing in order to feed your body more life-lengthening and youth-giving oxygen. So that your face gets its fair share of rejuvenation, you will also learn how to incorporate Fantastic Faces with every Synergetics motion. These funny faces can prevent or flex away a double chin, deep lines, and wrinkles. Fantastic Faces can help get rid of stress and depression. You will also learn Leg Synergetics which can resculpture your legs and behind if you incorporate them into your twice daily exercise routine.

Note! All photographs show the mirror image of what you are doing. So when the instructions say pull or push to your right, that means pull or push to *your* right!

Congratulations! You are about to begin creating your new self!

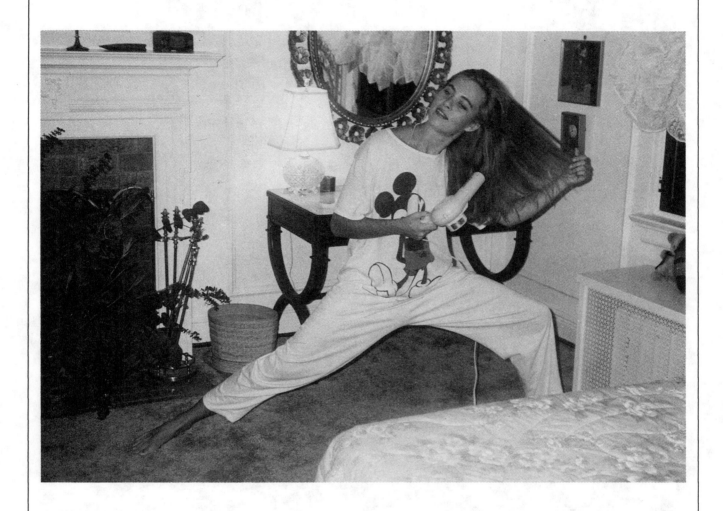

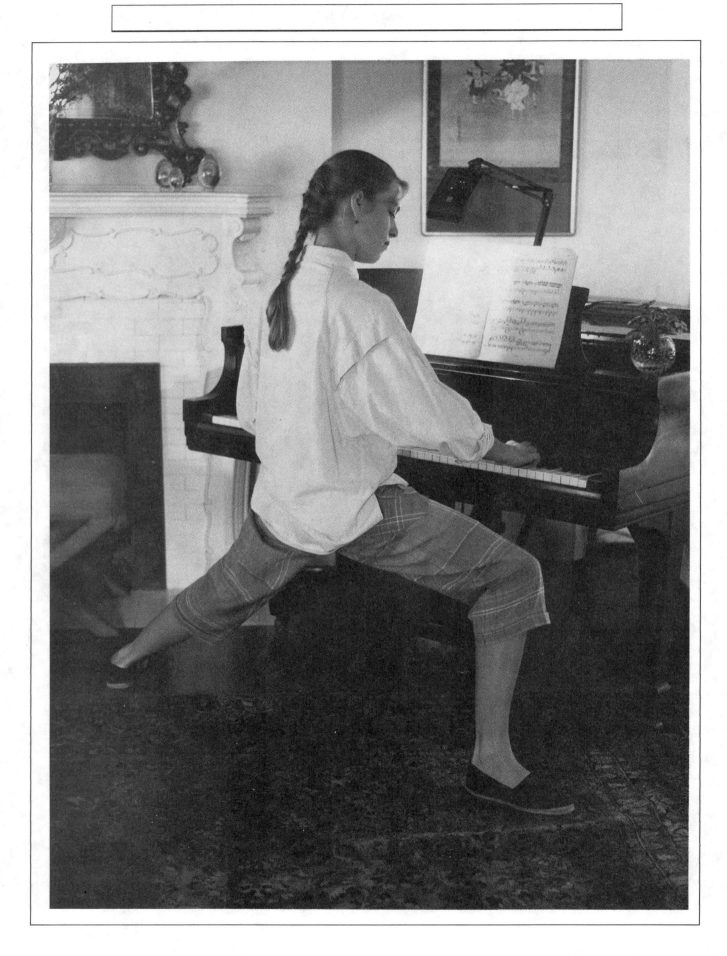

4

Basic Rainbows
Week One

The following pages contain the complete program for your first week. The instructions for the exercises follow in the order they are introduced in the program. Each workout will take approximately 12 minutes if you work straight through the program without stopping.

One Chest-High Pull is a complete back and forth motion (to the right and to the left), taking approximately 4 seconds total (2 seconds to the right, 2 seconds to the left). Count, one thousand one, one thousand two to the right, and one thousand three, one thousand four to the left.

Ten Weight Shifts means practicing weight shifting (that you learned in Chapter 3) and deep breathing back and forth 10 times. *Ten Chest-High Pulls and Pushes* means do 10 Pulls and 10 Pushes. When the words *Pulls and Pushes* are reversed *(Pushes and Pulls),* do the Pushes first.

For the first few days your programs will not require the entire 12 minutes. This extra time gives you a chance to stop and review from time to time. In the final days of the first week and through the second week, every second (all 720 of them) will be used up with a Synergetics exercise. Assuming you do your Synergetics motions at the Basic Tempo (4 seconds) you will do 180 repetitions (360 flexes) per workout, 720 flexes a day, 5,040 a week! A little bit a day adds up to a beautifully conditioned body.

On Day Five, you will be introduced to Fantastic Faces. From that day on, practice Fantastic Faces with every Rainbow you do.

DAY ONE

MORNING

Do in sequence:

10 Weight Shifts
10 Chest-High Pulls and Pushes
Repeat the above two more times

EVENING

Do in sequence:

10 Chest-High Pushes and Pulls
10 Weight Shifts
Repeat the above two more times

DAY TWO

MORNING

Do in sequence:

10 Chest-High Pulls and Pushes
10 Weight Shifts
10 Low Pulls and Pushes
5 Weight Shifts
Repeat the above one more time

EVENING

Do in sequence:

5 Weight Shifts
10 Low Pushes and Pulls
10 Weight Shifts
10 Chest-High Pushes and Pulls
Repeat the above one more time

DAY THREE

MORNING

Do in sequence:

10 Overhead Pulls and Pushes
10 Low Pulls and Pushes
10 Chest-High Pulls and Pushes
Repeat the above one more time

EVENING

Do in sequence:

10 Chest-High Pushes and Pulls
10 Overhead Pushes and Pulls
10 Low Pushes and Pulls
Repeat the above one more time

DAY FOUR

MORNING

Do in sequence:

10 Behind-The-Back Pulls and Pushes
10 Low Pulls and Pushes
10 Chest-High Pulls and Pushes
5 Overhead Pulls and Pushes
Repeat the above one more time

EVENING

Do in sequence:

10 Overhead Pushes and Pulls
5 Chest-High Pushes and Pulls
10 Low Pushes and Pulls
10 Behind-The-Back Pushes and Pulls
Repeat the above one more time

DAY FIVE

Fantastic Faces! They'll make you smile, they'll make you laugh, and they'll make you look younger and younger every day. They'll chase away miserable feelings, stress, and depression. Read the section on Fantastic Faces.

| **MORNING** | **EVENING** |
Do in sequence:	Do in sequence:
10 of each **Basic** Rainbow in the order you learned them	10 of each **Basic** Rainbow in the reverse order you learned them
Include all four of the Fantastic Faces in your program from now on	Continue to do Fantastic Faces with every Rainbow
Repeat the above one more time	Repeat the above one more time

DAY SIX

Carefully study and practice the section on Power Breathing. Use Power Breathing with every motion from now on.

| **MORNING** | **EVENING** |
Do in sequence:	Do in sequence:
10 of each **Basic** Rainbow in reverse order	10 of each **Basic** Rainbow in order
Incorporate a Fantastic Face and Power Breathing with every Rainbow	Incorporate a Fantastic Face and Power Breathing with every Rainbow
Repeat the above one more time	Repeat the above one more time

DAY SEVEN

Today is review day. A review of you. How do you feel? Stronger? More relaxed? More energetic? Do you see subtle changes in your appearance when you look in the mirror? Is it becoming easier for you to stand up straighter? Take this day and invest your two 12-minute workouts in practicing the Rainbows that you feel need the most work. And practice, practice, practice Power Breathing. Don't forget Fantastic Faces!

By the end of this first week, you'll have a good feel for Synergetics. You'll also be forming a lifetime habit of exercise. Now on to the instructions!

BASIC CHEST-HIGH PULL

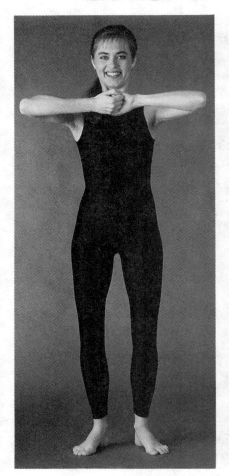 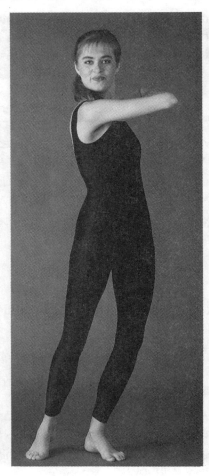 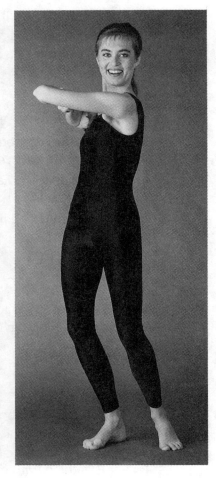

1

Stand with your heels 6" apart, feet angled out. Hook your fingers together. Hold your hands and elbows at shoulder level with your elbows bent at right angles. Tuck your hips forward, so it feels as though your hips are positioned under your shoulders. Smile!

2

Inhale deeply as you slowly pull your hands with steady force to your right. Keep your left elbow locked at a right angle. Remember to hold your arms at shoulder level. Shift your weight to the ball of your right foot. Be sure to keep your knees slightly bent with your hips tucked under. Hold your head high and straight forward.

3

Exhale completely as you slowly pull your hands with steady force back to your left. Keep your right elbow locked at a right angle. Remember to hold your arms at shoulder level. Shift your weight to the ball of your left foot. Allow your hips to follow. Pull your body gently into a tight twist. Stand tall, chin in. Continue back to your right and repeat.

BASIC CHEST-HIGH PUSH

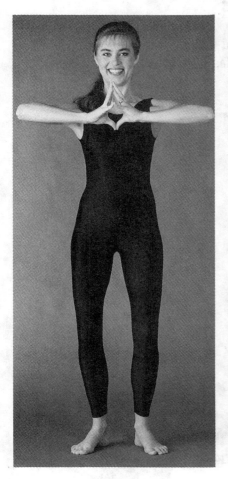 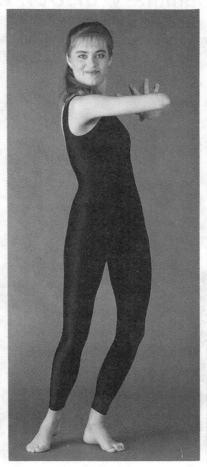 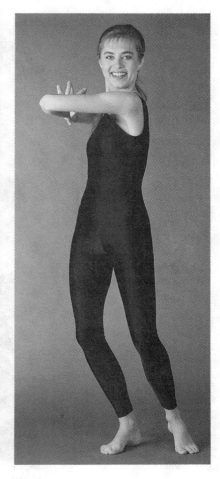

1

Stand with your heels 6" apart, feet angled out and knees slightly bent. Press the tips of your fingers and thumbs together with your elbows bent at right angles. Hold your hands and elbows at shoulder level. Smile!

2

Inhale deeply as you slowly push your hands with steady force to your right. Keep your left elbow locked at a right angle. Remember to hold your arms at shoulder level. Shift your weight to the ball of your right foot. Push your body gently into a tight twist. Don't push so hard that the motion is jerky or shaky. Stand tall, chin in.

3

Exhale completely as you slowly push your hands with steady force back to your left. Keep your right elbow locked at a right angle. Remember to hold your arms at shoulder level. Shift your weight to the ball of your left foot. Let your hands push your body into a gentle left twist. Allow your hips to follow. Hold your head high and straight forward. Keep your hips tucked under. Continue back to your right and repeat.

POOR POSTURE
Summary of Don'ts

This picture is not a complete exaggeration! Look around you as you go through your day and you'll probably see some people standing this way. Don't be one of them!

DO NOT

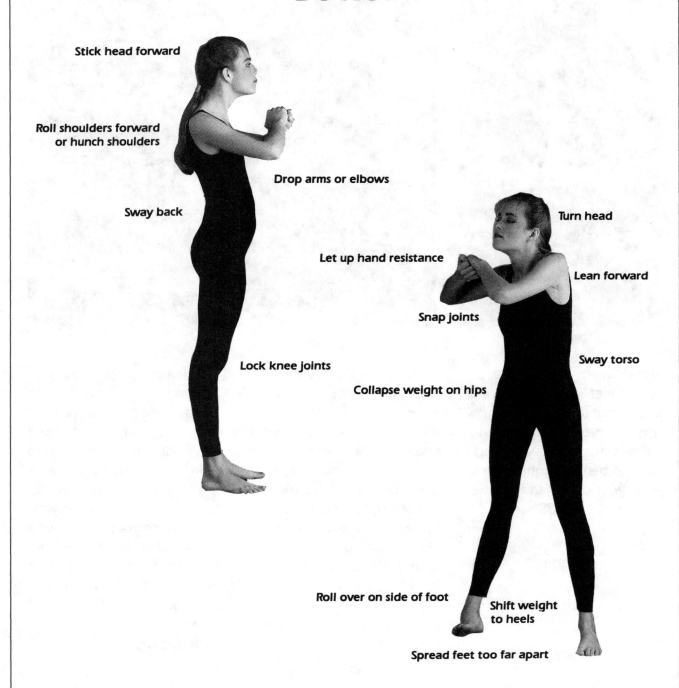

Stick head forward

Roll shoulders forward
or hunch shoulders

Sway back

Drop arms or elbows

Turn head

Let up hand resistance

Lean forward

Snap joints

Lock knee joints

Sway torso

Collapse weight on hips

Roll over on side of foot

Shift weight
to heels

Spread feet too far apart

PERFECT POSTURE
Summary of Do's

By standing correctly with Perfect Posture, as you do Synergetics, you can develop more strength in the muscles that hold your body straight naturally. Think about your posture while you work out, and your muscles will develop to help you hold your body beautifully straight.

DO

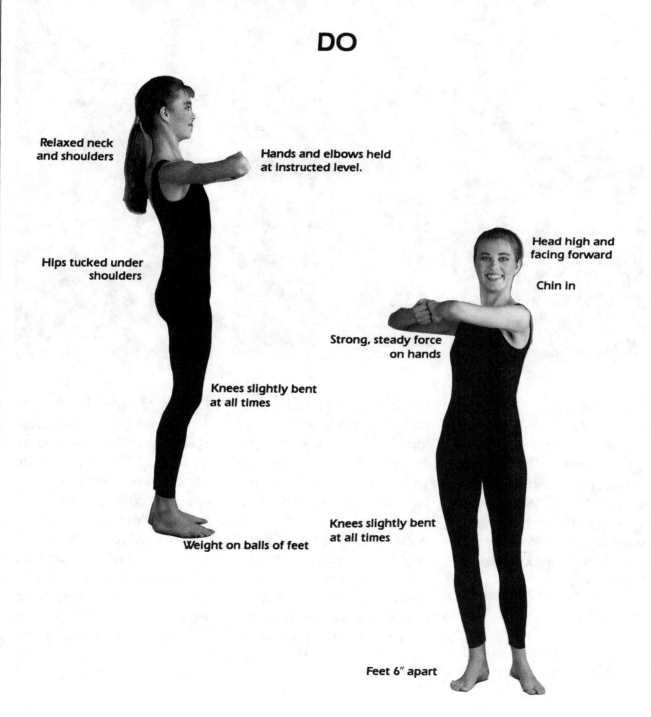

Relaxed neck and shoulders

Hands and elbows held at instructed level.

Hips tucked under shoulders

Head high and facing forward

Chin in

Strong, steady force on hands

Knees slightly bent at all times

Knees slightly bent at all times

Weight on balls of feet

Feet 6″ apart

BASIC LOW PULL

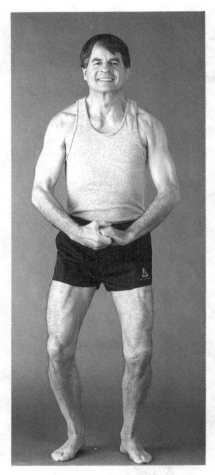 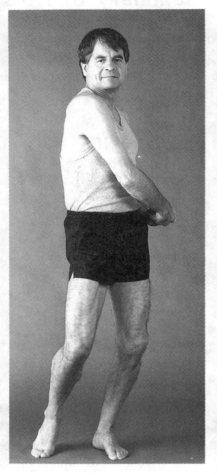 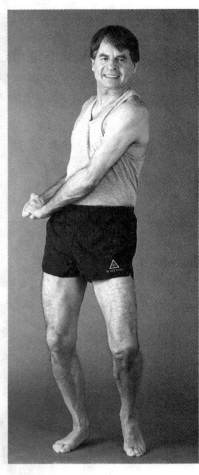

1

Stand with your heels 6" apart, feet angled out and knees slightly bent. Hook your fingers 6" below your bellybutton. Bend your elbows slightly. Stand with your weight on the balls of your feet and don't rock your weight back onto your heels. Smile!

2

Inhale deeply as you slowly pull your hands with steady force around to your right. Try to pull your hands into your imaginary right hip pocket. Shift your weight to the ball of your right foot. Allow your hips to follow, gently pulling your body into a right twist. Hold your hands low and close to your body throughout the motion. Hold your head high and straight forward.

3

Exhale completely as you slowly pull your hands with steady force back around to your left. Try to pull your hands into your imaginary left hip pocket. Shift your weight to the ball of your left foot. Allow your hips to follow. Don't pull so hard that the motion is jerky or shaky. Stand tall, chin in. Keep your hips tucked under. Continue back to your right and repeat.

BASIC LOW PUSH

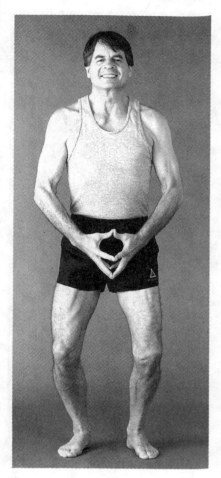 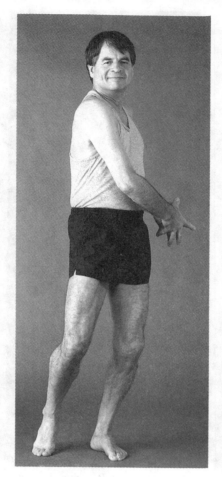 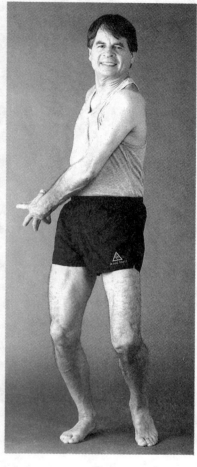

1

Stand with your heels 6" apart, feet angled out and knees slightly bent. Press the tips of your fingers and thumbs together 6" below your bellybutton. Bend your elbows slightly. Stand tall, chin in. Smile!

2

Inhale deeply as you slowly push your hands with steady force to your right. Try to push your hands into your imaginary right hip pocket. Shift your weight to the ball of your right foot as you gently push your body into a tight right twist. The Basic Tempo is two counts to the right. Hold your head high and straight forward.

3

Exhale completely as you slowly push your hands with steady force back to your left. Try to push your hands into your imaginary left hip pocket. Shift your weight to the ball of your left foot as you gently push your body into a tight left twist. The Basic Tempo is two counts to the left. Hold your head high and straight forward. Continue back to your right and repeat.

BASIC OVERHEAD PULL

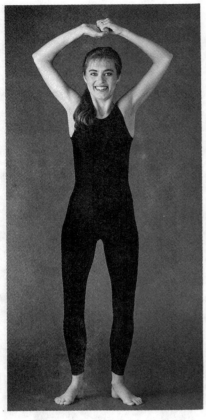

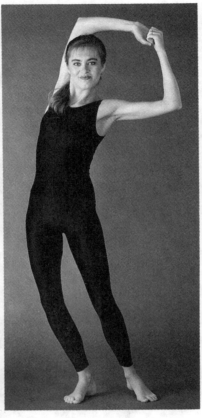

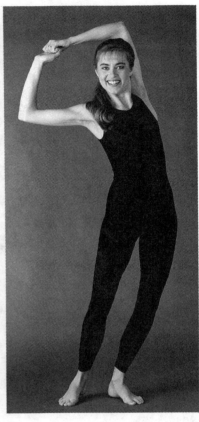

1

Stand with your heels 6" apart, feet angled out. Hook your fingers together 3" over your head. Pull your hands and elbows toward the back of your head as far as you can. Lock your elbows at right angles. Be sure your shoulders are relaxed. Smile!

2

Inhale deeply as you slowly pull your hands with steady force over your right shoulder. Remember to keep your hands and elbows back and your elbows locked at the same right angles that you started with. Shift your weight to the ball of your left foot, keeping your knees slightly bent. Allow your hips to sway to your left. Bend your body only as far as you can without dropping your head to the side. Hold your head high and straight forward.

3

Exhale completely as you slowly pull your hands with steady force back over your head, over your left shoulder. Remember to keep your hands and elbows back and your elbows locked at the same right angles that you started with in Step 1. Shift your weight to the ball of your right foot. Allow your hips to sway to your right. Keep in mind that you are shifting your weight to the opposite foot from which you are pulling your hands. Continue back to your right and repeat.

BASIC OVERHEAD PUSH

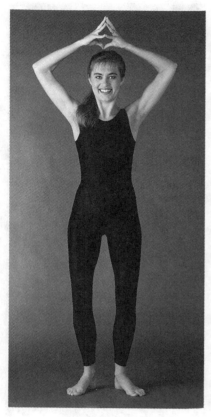

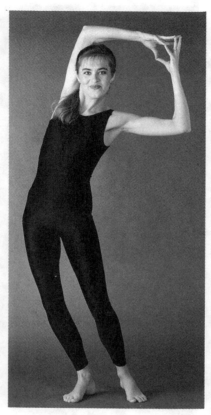

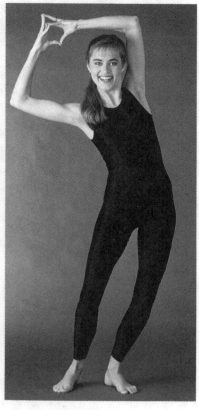

1

Stand with your heels 6" apart, feet angled out. Press the tips of your fingers and thumbs together 3" over your head. Push your hands and elbows toward the rear of your head as far as you can. Lock your elbows at right angles. Be sure to keep your knees slightly bent throughout the following motion. Smile!

2

Inhale deeply as you slowly push your hands with steady force over your right shoulder. Remember to keep your hands and elbows back and your elbows locked at the same right angle that you started with. Shift your weight to the ball of your left foot. Allow your hips to sway to your left. Concentrate on inhaling all the way across the motion. Stand tall, chin in.

3

Exhale completely as you slowly push your hands with steady force back over your head, over your left shoulder. Remember to keep your hands and elbows back and your elbows locked at the same right angle that you started with in Step 1. Shift your weight to the ball of your right foot. Allow your hips to sway to your right. Don't bend your body any farther than you can while keeping your head straight up. Continue back to your right and repeat.

BASIC BEHIND-THE-BACK PULL

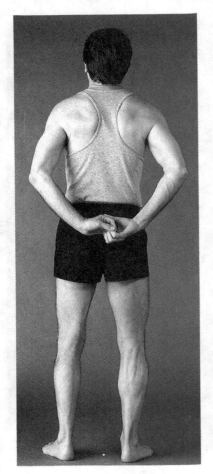

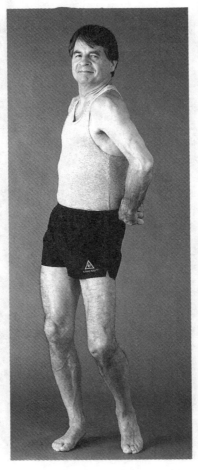

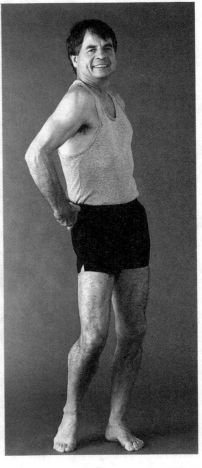

1

Stand with your heels 6" apart, feet angled out. Hook your fingers together behind your back at the bottom of your spine. Bend your elbows slightly. Stand with Perfect Posture. Smile!

2

Inhale deeply as you slowly pull your hands with steady force to your right. Try to pull your hands into your imaginary right front pocket. Concentrate on pointing your right elbow forward for a better flex. Shift your weight to the ball of your left foot while keeping your knees slightly bent. Hold your head high and straight forward.

3

Exhale completely as you slowly pull your hands with steady force back to your left. Try to pull your hands into your imaginary left front pocket. Concentrate on pointing your left elbow forward for a better flex. Shift your weight to the ball of your right foot. Don't let your weight collapse onto your right hip. Stand tall, chin in. Keep in mind that you shift your weight to the opposite foot from which you are pulling your hands. Continue back to your right and repeat.

BASIC BEHIND-THE-BACK PUSH

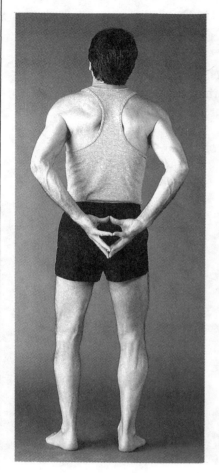 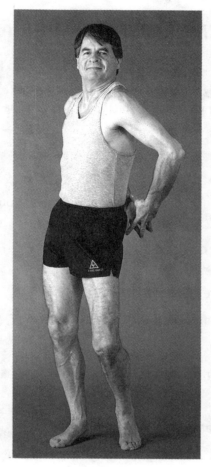 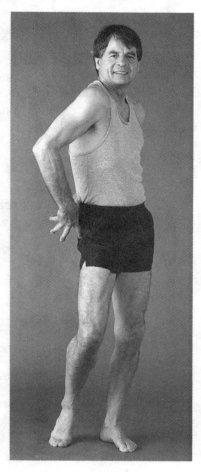

1

Stand with your heels 6" apart, feet angled out and your knees slightly bent. Press the tips of your fingers and thumbs together behind your back at the bottom of your spine. Bend your elbows slightly. Relax your shoulders. Smile!

2

Inhale deeply as you slowly push your hands with steady force to your right. Try to push your hands into your imaginary right front pocket. Concentrate on pointing your right elbow forward for a good flex. Shift your weight to the ball of your left foot. Don't allow your foot to roll over on its side as you shift your weight. Hold your head high and straight forward.

3

Exhale completely as you slowly push your hands with steady force back to your left. Try to push your hands into your imaginary left front pocket. Concentrate on pointing your left elbow forward for a good flex. Shift your weight to the ball of your right foot. Let your hands push your body into a gentle twist. Stand tall, chin in. Continue back to your right and repeat.

SYNERGETICS FEELINGS

Here is a checklist of positive sensations and changes which you should begin to experience after doing Synergetics twice a day for a while. If there are any particular feelings or sensations in your body which concern you, be sure to consult with your physician.

	CHECK ONE	
	YES	NO
Do you feel your spine and neck pleasantly flexing as you pull or push into a sway or a twist?	_____	_____
Do you feel your thigh, calf, and buttock muscles tighten on the side where you shift your weight?	_____	_____
Do you feel that you are breathing more deeply?	_____	_____
Do you feel energized after your Synergetics workouts?	_____	_____
Do you feel growing sensations in your muscle fibers?	_____	_____
Do you feel your heart rate increase as you work out?	_____	_____
Do you feel stronger?	_____	_____
Do you feel more calm after a set of Synergetics?	_____	_____
Do you feel that you are standing up straighter, walking taller?	_____	_____
Do you feel that you are sleeping better?	_____	_____
Do you feel yourself getting more grace and balance?	_____	_____

The more conscious you are of your positive changes, the more you will enjoy them.

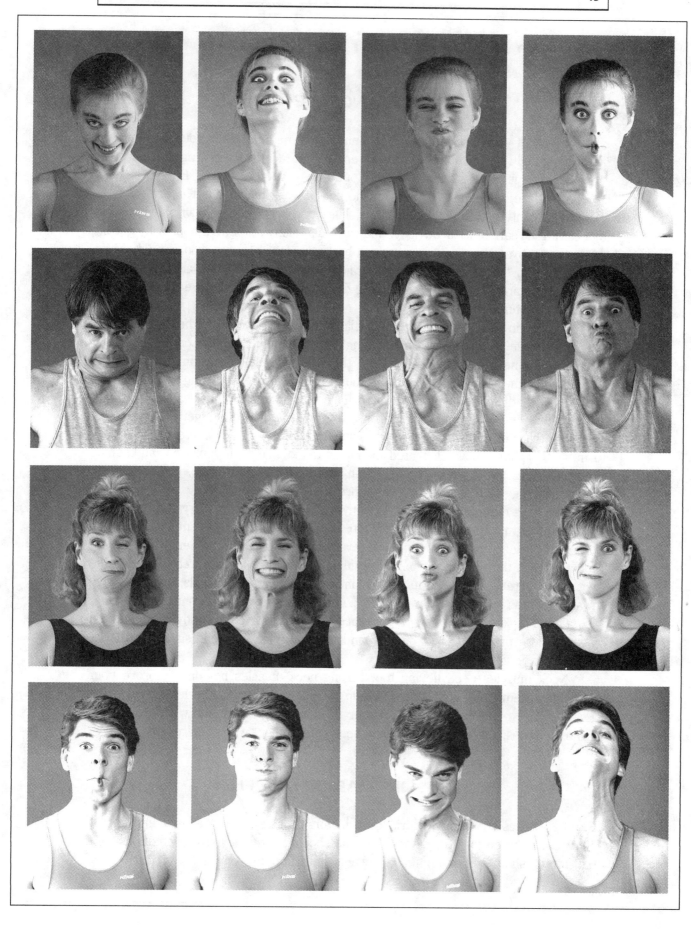

FANTASTIC FACES

SAVING FACE

The beauty of your face is more than skin deep. The muscles in your face must be kept beautifully toned too. You can rejuvenate your face by exercising those sagging muscles that pull your skin and features out of their youthful shape. Even at an early age, your face will begin to sag from the pull of slack muscles if it doesn't get the proper amount of flexing. Double chins, lines in the cheeks, and wrinkled lips can appear after years of facial atrophy. You can make many of them disappear by getting your face active. Have you ever noticed how your face appears to droop when you first get up in the morning? This is because it has had no flexing all night. If your face muscles aren't exercised during the day, it won't be long before they will begin to sag all the time.

Contracting and expanding the facial muscles will activate the thousands of sagging muscle fibers in your face, making it supple and beautifully contoured. There has been some argument that flexing the face wrinkles the skin. Much of the wrinkling of the skin comes from the muscles in the face shrinking from **atrophy** (which allows the skin to sag), or from **only contracting** the muscles like frowning, or wrinkling the lips while taking a drag from a cigarette. Synergetics face flexing requires that you *contract* and *expand* your facial muscles, just like exercising your arm, so that they remain elongated and highly toned, filling out your skin and keeping it pliable. You can fill out your saggy skin with newly toned muscle, just as you can fill up the saggy skin of a balloon with more air.

Skin cells die from lack of oxygen (hypoxia) and lack of capillary stimulation, as well as drying out from lack of water, too much sun, and cigarette smoke. Flex your face every day and breathe deeply with every breath. Use a sunscreen when you are going to be in the sun for any period of time. You might also want to be aware of the fact that cigarette smoke coats your skin with face-aging chemicals, so try to stay away from it as much as you can. Drink plenty of water every day, and after bathing, use a good moisturizing lotion on your face and over your entire body. If you are on a weight loss program, facial flexing can keep your skin tight and supple as the fat melts from your face.

Neck muscles need flexing too. Strong neck muscles not only improve your looks, complementing your face, but help your posture and the health of your spine as well. The more you can make your neck muscles stick out when you make Fantastic Faces, the less your chin and neck will hang out when you're not.

THE THREE-MARTINI FACE FLEX

Facial exercises are being prescribed by doctors for stress management. In everyday life, we are forced to repress the faces that should accompany strong emotions—we try not to show our emotions. So stress gets into the entire body. As a quick experiment, right now, look in the mirror, make your best "You can't make me!" face and stick out your tongue. Did you feel that release? That's the key to getting a stress release any time you feel like it.

THE MOST FANTASTIC FACE OF ALL

There is one face you can do all day long, but you may attract a lot of attention! Some people will just stare wistfully at you—wishing they felt like you do—but many will return your Fantastic Face with one of their own. What is it? Your best and warmest Smile! It's a universal signal that you feel good, that you are friendly, and that you want to share your good feelings. Notice how people watch you when you're smiling. Try it! The next time you're in the grocery store or shopping mall by yourself, just go around smiling and notice how you seem to light up all of the people around you. And be conscious of how good you feel inside as your eyes sparkle and your face glows with energy. That's right, energy!

So smile at everything and with everything! Life really is fun (and funny) if you're feeling good. Let your smile peek through the Fantastic Faces, and your whole being will fill with smiles. Remember, the funnier face you can make during Synergetics time, the more beautiful your face will be all the time.

Every morning and every evening you can give yourself a 12-minute face lift. The Hunter, Popeye, and Guppy are particularly good for preventing or getting rid of wrinkles on your cheeks and lips, and the Gorilla is very good for getting rid of a double chin and toning all of your neck muscles. Why not have a youthful face to match your youthful body?

THE HUNTER

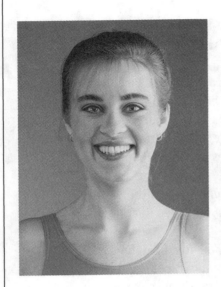

1

Face forward and smile.

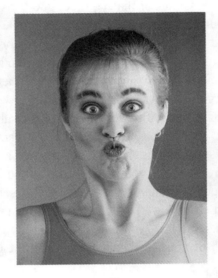

2

Deeply inhale through your nose, bug your eyes, and purse your lips as hard as you can. Don't clench your teeth. Hold your head back, don't jut your head forward. Hold this expression all the way through the inhale.

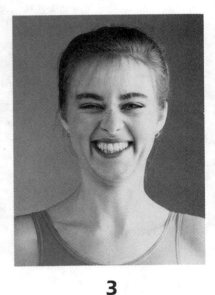

3

Completely exhale from your mouth, squint your eyes, and push your lips back from your teeth into a cheek-tightening smile. Hold this expression all the way through your exhale.

THE POPEYE

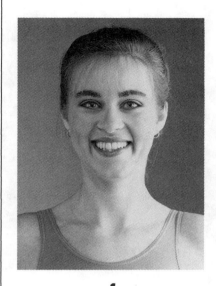

1

Face forward and smile.

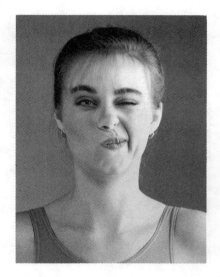

2

Deeply inhale through your nose, pull your lips as far as you can to your right, and squint your right eye. (Move your jaw as little as possible.) Hold this expression all the way through your inhale.

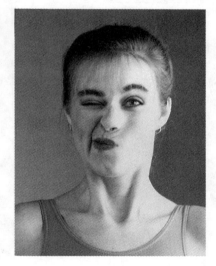

3

Completely exhale from your mouth, pull your lips as far as you can to your left, and squint your left eye. (Move your jaw as little as possible.) Hold this expression all the way through your exhale. For the best stretch, always pull your mouth in the opposite direction from which you are pulling or pushing your hands.

THE GUPPY

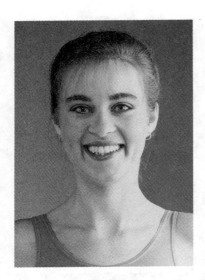

1

Face forward and smile.

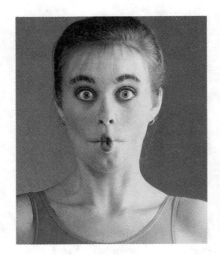

2

Deeply inhale through your nose, bug your eyes, open your jaw, and suck your cheeks in between your teeth. Hold this expression all the way through your inhale.

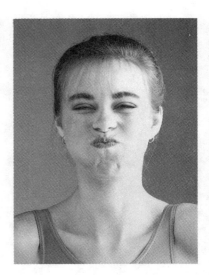

3

Completely exhale from your nose, squint your eyes, puff out your cheeks, and close your jaw. Hold this expression all the way through your exhale. Don't clench your teeth.

THE GORILLA

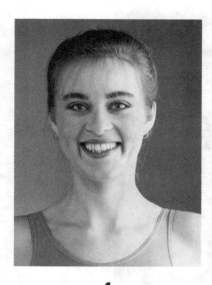

1

Face forward and smile. (Be prepared for your chin and neck muscles to feel a little sore for the first few days.)

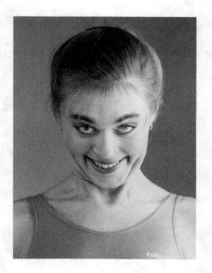

2

Deeply inhale through your nose, drop your relaxed chin to your chest. Then make a cheek-tightening smile as hard as you can and hold it. Fix your eyes on a spot straight ahead.

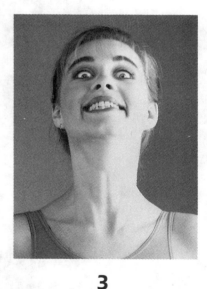

3

Completely exhale from your mouth, hold the cheek-tightening smile and slowly rock your head back as far as you can. Keep your eyes fixed on that same spot. Don't clench your teeth. Repeat steps two and three.

COMBINING FANTASTIC

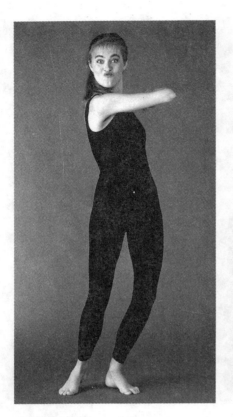

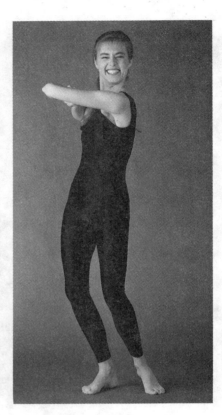

The Hunter

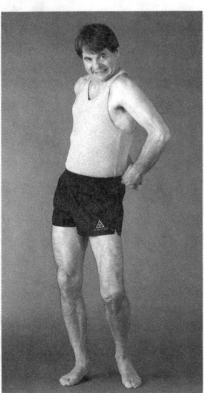

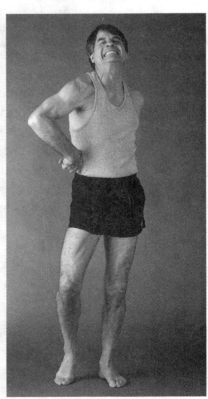

The Gorilla

FACES WITH RAINBOWS

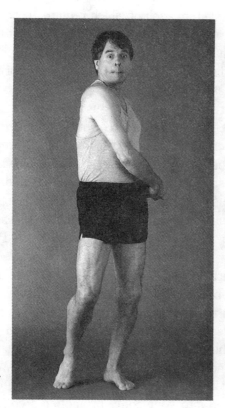
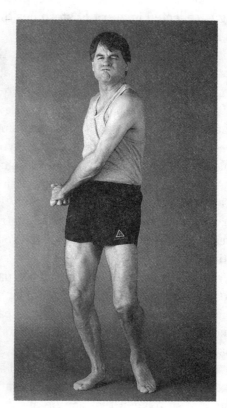

The Guppy

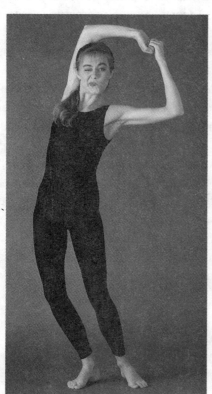
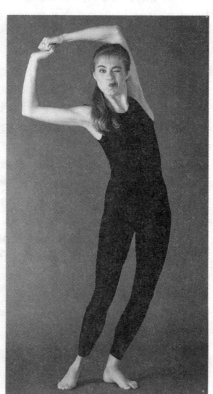

The Popeye

THE ART OF POWER BREATHING

"Life is in the breath, therefore he who only half breathes, half lives." This Yogic saying is reflected in every Eastern health system each of which requires complete, conscious breathing in order to energize, balance, and heal the body. We must teach our bodies how to absorb more oxygen than normal, to help keep us from prematurely aging. Your goal with Power Breathing is to train your body to absorb the optimum amount of oxygen with every breath.

It's easy to demonstrate how Power Breathing works, because you automatically go through the action every day without knowing it. Place your hands on your stomach. Now, cough. Did you feel your stomach muscles extend before you coughed, and then contract as you coughed? Now try a sneeze, a nose blow, or a laugh. The action that your stomach just took (expanding as you inhaled, and contracting as you exhaled) is probably just the opposite of the way you do your normal breathing (unless you've been trained in singing or in Eastern breathing techniques). These are the motions you must practice in order to learn Power Breathing.

Most of us breathe with the upper part of our lungs only. Using only the upper part of your lungs limits the amount of air you can take in because the lung expansion is limited by your rib cage. The lower parts of your lungs have more flexibility to expand. But they are often partially constricted because most people hold their stomach muscles in instead of allowing the stomach muscles to relax so that the lower part of the lungs can freely expand and take in a full amount of oxygen. We call this restrictive type of breathing, Starvation Breathing. Starvation Breathing limits the amount of oxygen that can be absorbed into your body, promoting a condition called hypoxia (too little oxygen to the cells) which causes premature aging of the body.

Breathe by extending your stomach as you inhale, allowing your lower lungs to fill with air first, and then continue to inhale by filling your upper lungs with air. Then contract your stomach muscles as you exhale, to expel as much spent air as possible. This will dramatically increase the quantity of oxygen you take in with every breath. It will enhance your health, increase your energy, strengthen your stomach muscles, and trim your waist.

At first, breathing this way may seem strange and confusing to your body, since you may have already taken over a half billion shallow Starvation Breaths in your life. Practice Power Breathing with every Synergetics motion. Practice it whenever you can: watching television, reading a book, working at your desk. It is a great stress chaser and in time, this natural method of breathing will become the way you breathe all the time. When the instructions say, *inhale deeply* or *exhale completely,* that means Power Breathing. No more shallow Starvation Breathing!

POWER BREATHING

INHALE

INHALE

EXHALE

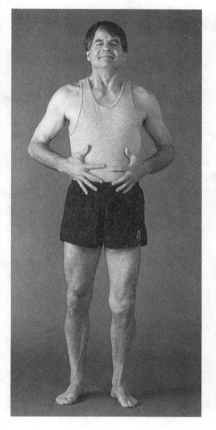

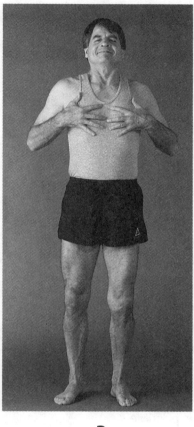

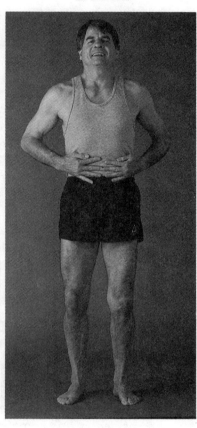

1

Stand tall with your hands on your stomach, so you can feel the muscles expand. Inhale slowly through your nose. As you inhale, relax your abdominal muscles and expand your stomach, filling your lower lungs with air. Try to make your stomach stick out as far as you can.

2

Still inhaling, pull more air in to allow your upper lungs (chest cavity) to fill with air. Move your hands up to your chest and feel it expand. Filling your lungs with air is like filling a glass with water— you do it from the bottom up.

3

Now exhale from your open mouth by contracting your stomach muscles. Put your hands back on your stomach and feel the muscles contract. Pull your stomach in toward your backbone and force all the old air out of your open mouth. Don't purse your lips and constrict the air exit, let your lips and jaw relax. Make a soft ''aaaaahhh'' sound as the air escapes. Really feel the stomach action. Practice until you can do Power Breathing with a natural, easy rhythm.

PERFECT FORM CHECKLIST

As you go through the Synergetics motions, be sure that your body is following the proper form, so you get maximum benefits from your workouts.

	CHECK ONE	
	YES	**NO**
Are you smiling?	_____	_____
Are you holding your head high and facing forward?	_____	_____
Are you Power Breathing—expanding and contracting your stomach muscles?	_____	_____
Are you doing a Fantastic Face?	_____	_____
Are you keeping your chin tucked?	_____	_____
Are you pulling and pushing with constant force and speed?	_____	_____
Are you developing a smooth, consistent rhythm?	_____	_____
Are you holding your hands and elbows at the correct level?	_____	_____
Are you coming to a gentle stop without jerking?	_____	_____
Are you holding your elbows locked at the instructed angle?	_____	_____
Are you pulling and pushing with enough resistance?	_____	_____
Are you giving yourself enough time to inhale and exhale as deeply and completely as possible?	_____	_____
Are you pulling and pushing your body to the maximum without ducking or turning your head?	_____	_____
Are you keeping your hips tucked under your shoulders?	_____	_____
Are you keeping your weight from collapsing on your hips?	_____	_____
Are you gently twisting your body without swaying your hips?	_____	_____
Are you shifting your weight to the proper foot?	_____	_____
Are you keeping your knees slightly bent?	_____	_____
Are you keeping your heels 6" apart, toes turned outward?	_____	_____
Are you shifting your weight completely from one foot to the other?	_____	_____

BRAINSTORMS AND ENERGY BURSTS

YOUR PERSONAL PROGRESS RECORD

DATE	WEIGHT	WAIST	HIPS	THIGHS	CHEST	STRENGTH (1–10)

COORDINATION (1–10)	ENERGY (1–10)	RELAXED (1–10)	SLEEP (1–10)

ELIMINATION (1–10)	EATING HABITS (1–10)	FACE (1–10)	OVERALL APPEARANCE (1–10)

OVERALL FEELINGS (1–10)   NOTE: Score 1 as low and 10 as high.

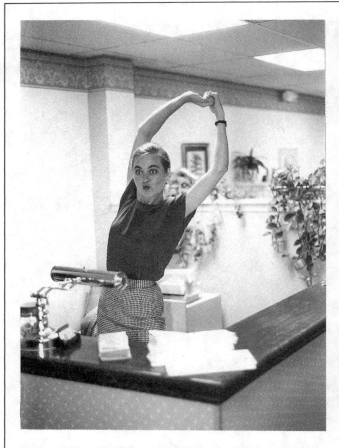
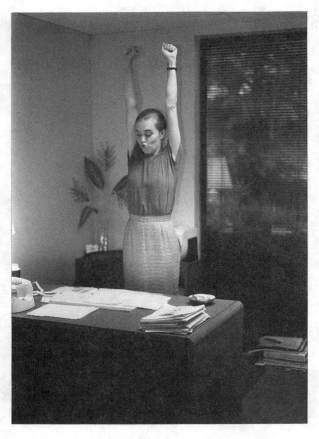
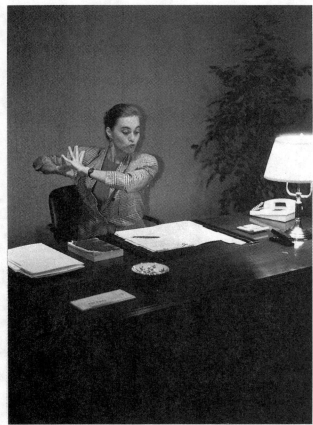
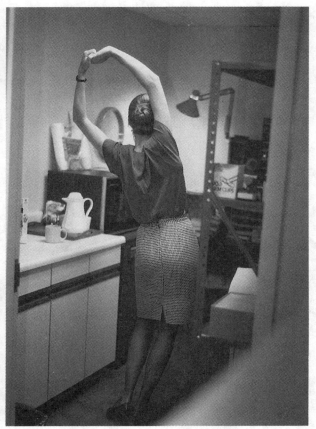

5

Extended Rainbows and Leg Synergetics
Week Two

Congratulations! You have graduated to the next level—Extended Rainbows and Leg Synergetics! These exercises will challenge your mind and body just like the Basic Rainbows did—calling on new muscle combinations, and developing more functional strength and body contour. Always include Power Breathing and Fantastic Faces with every Rainbow you do. The results will be well worth your extra effort. Remember that all photographs are intended to be your mirror image.

DAY ONE

MORNING

Do in sequence:

10 Extended Chest-High Pulls and Pushes

5 of each **Basic** Rainbow in order

10 Extended Chest-High Pulls and Pushes

Repeat the above one more time

EVENING

Do in sequence:

10 Extended Chest-High Pushes and Pulls

5 of each **Basic** Rainbow in reverse order

10 Extended Chest-High Pushes and Pulls

Repeat the above one more time

DAY TWO

MORNING

Do in sequence:

10 Extended Low Pulls and Pushes

5 Extended Chest-High Pulls and Pushes

5 of each **Basic** Rainbow in order

5 Extended Low Pulls and Pushes

5 Extended Chest-High Pulls and Pushes

Repeat the above one more time

EVENING

Do in sequence:

5 Extended Chest-High Pushes and Pulls

5 Extended Low Pushes and Pulls

5 of each **Basic** Rainbow in reverse order

5 Extended Chest-High Pushes and Pulls

10 Extended Low Pushes and Pulls

Repeat the above one more time

DAY THREE

MORNING
Do in sequence:

10 Extended Overhead Pulls
and Pushes

5 Extended Chest-High Pulls
and Pushes

5 Extended Low Pulls and Pushes

5 of each **Basic** Rainbow in order

5 Extended Overhead Pulls
and Pushes

Repeat the above one more time

EVENING
Do in sequence:

5 Extended Overhead Pushes
and Pulls

5 of each **Basic** Rainbow in
reverse order

5 Extended Low Pushes and Pulls

5 Extended Chest-High Pushes
and Pulls

10 Extended Overhead Pushes
and Pulls

Repeat the above one more time

DAY FOUR

MORNING
Do in sequence:

10 Extended Behind-the-Back Pulls
and Pushes

5 Extended Low Pulls and Pushes

5 Extended Chest-High Pulls
and Pushes

5 Extended Overhead Pulls
and Pushes

5 of each **Basic** Rainbow in order

Repeat the above one more time

EVENING
Do in sequence:

5 of each **Basic** Rainbow in order

5 Extended Overhead Pushes
and Pulls

5 Extended Chest-High Pushes
and Pulls

5 Extended Low Pushes and Pulls

10 Extended Behind-the-Back Pushes
and Pulls

Repeat the above one more time

DAY FIVE

Practice the Cat Stretch. *20 Cat Stretches* means do 20 Cat Stretches up and down.

MORNING	**EVENING**
Do in sequence:	Do in sequence:

20 Cat Stretches	5 of each **Extended** Rainbow in reverse order
5 of each **Extended** Rainbow in order	5 of each **Basic** Rainbow in reverse order
5 of each **Basic** Rainbow in order	20 Cat Stretches
Repeat the above one more time	Repeat the above one more time

DAY SIX

Read and practice Stepping Out. Your legs are getting a very good workout just by Weight Shifts and Cat Stretches, but when you add Stepping Out to your program, your legs and buttocks will take on even more beautiful dimensions and tone.

MORNING	**EVENING**
Do in sequence:	Do in sequence:

15 Stepping Outs (right and left)	20 Cat Stretches
10 of each **Basic** Rainbow in order	10 of each **Extended** Rainbow in reverse order
5 of each **Extended** Rainbow in order	5 of each **Basic** Rainbow in reverse order
20 Cat Stretches	15 Stepping Outs (right and left)

DAY SEVEN

Read the section, Power Breathing Review.

Should you give your body a rest once a week? We have personally found that if we skip a day of Synergetics workouts, our bodies become a little depressed and lethargic. It's like skipping eating or not sleeping for a day. Our bodies need a proper balance of rest, food, and exercise to look young and feel energetic. So our recommendation is to always do some Synergetics, even if it is just part of a workout. That way you won't begin breaking a life-giving habit.

MORNING	EVENING
Do in sequence:	Do in sequence:
15 Stepping Outs (right and left)	10 of each **Extended** Rainbow Pushes and Pulls
10 of each **Basic** Rainbow Pulls and Pushes	10 of each **Basic** Rainbow Pushes and Pulls
10 of each **Extended** Rainbow Pulls and Pushes	15 Stepping Outs (right and left)

Once you have completed this second seven-day plan, you will have learned the Extended Rainbow series. Combined with the Basic Rainbows, this series will allow you to create your very own, very effective Synergetics workout. Now, on to the instructions!

EXTENDED CHEST-HIGH PULL

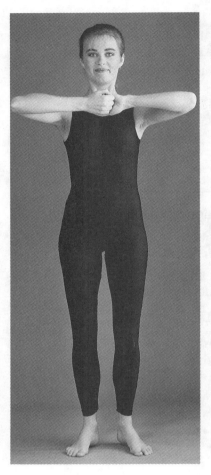

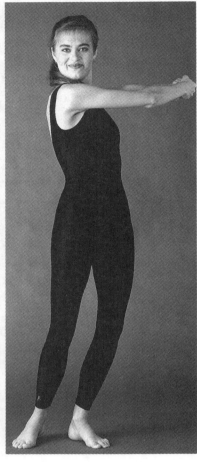

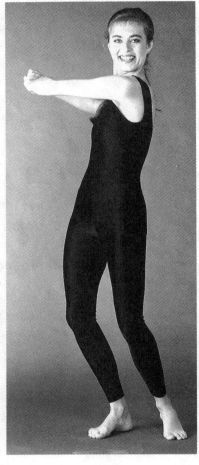

1

Stand with your heels 6″ apart, feet angled out and your knees slightly bent. Hook your fingers together. Extend your arms out in front of you at shoulder level. Bend your elbows slightly. Stand with Perfect Posture. Smile!

2

Inhale deeply as you slowly pull your hands with steady force to your right. Remember to hold your arms at shoulder level and keep your *left* elbow locked in the same, slightly bent position that you started with. Shift your weight to the ball of your right foot. Slowly pull your torso into a tight right twist. Make the motion very smooth and flowing. Hold your head high and straight forward.

3

Exhale completely as you slowly pull your hands with steady force back to your left. Remember to hold your arms at shoulder level and now keep your *right* elbow locked in the same, slightly bent position that you started with in Step 1. Shift your weight to the ball of your left foot. Pull your torso into a tight left twist. Keep in mind that you are shifting your weight to the same side as you are pulling your hands. Continue back to your right and repeat.

EXTENDED CHEST-HIGH PUSH

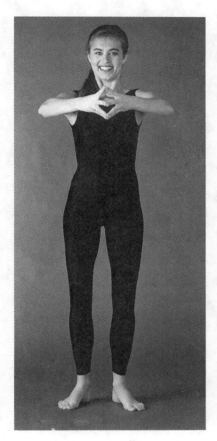

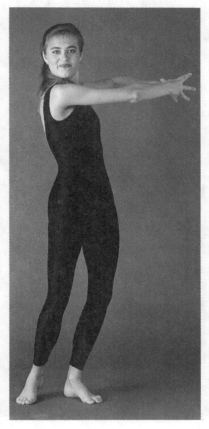

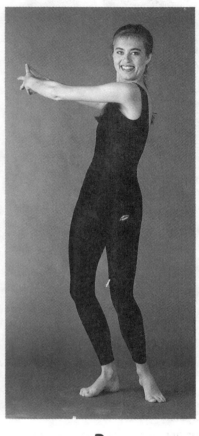

1

Stand with your heels 6" apart, feet angled out. Press the tips of your fingers and thumbs together. Extend your arms straight out in front of you at shoulder level. Bend your elbows slightly. Stand tall. Smile!

2

Inhale deeply as you slowly push your hands with steady force to your right. Remember to hold your arms at shoulder level and keep your *left* elbow locked in the same, slightly bent position that you started with. Shift your weight to the ball of your right foot, keeping your knees slightly bent. Don't sway—just push your body into a tight twist. Stand tall with your chin tucked in.

3

Exhale completely as you slowly push your hands with steady force back to your left. Remember to hold your arms at shoulder level and now keep your *right* elbow locked in that same, slightly bent position that you started with in Step 1. Shift your weight to the ball of your left foot. Allow your hips to follow. Concentrate on keeping your knees slightly bent and your hips tucked under. Continue back to your right and repeat.

EXTENDED LOW PULL

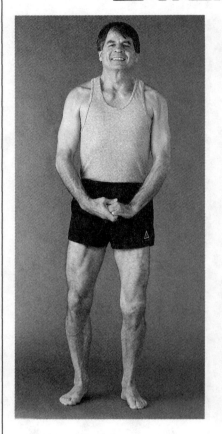 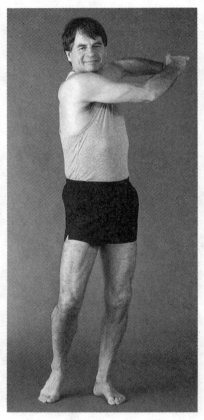 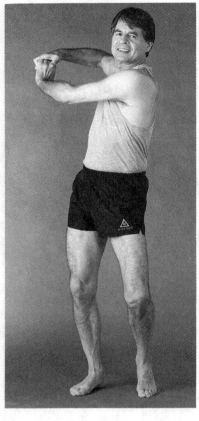

1

Stand with your heels 6" apart, feet angled out. Hook your fingers 6" below your bellybutton. Bend your elbows slightly. Smile!

2

Inhale deeply as you slowly pull your hands with steady force low and back to your right, then up to the height of your right shoulder. Remember to keep your *left* elbow locked in the same, slightly bent position that you started with. Shift your weight to the ball of your right foot. Be sure to keep your knees slightly bent with your hips tucked under at all times.

3

Exhale completely as you slowly pull your hands with steady force back down below your bellybutton. Keep your *left* elbow locked. With continuous motion pull your hands low and back to your left, then up to the height of your left shoulder, now keeping your *right* elbow locked in the same, slightly bent position that you started with in Step 1. Shift your weight to the ball of your left foot. Hold your head high and straight forward. Continue back to your right and repeat.

EXTENDED LOW PUSH

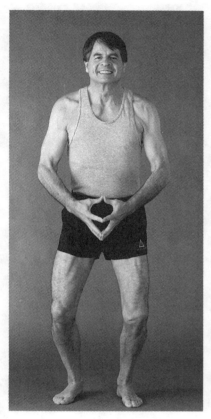

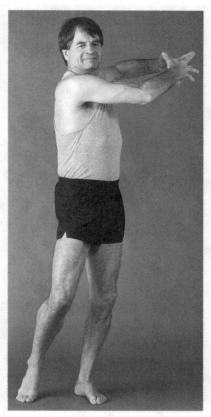

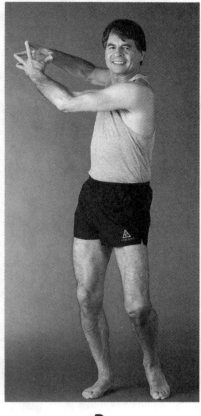

1

Stand with your heels 6" apart, feet angled out and knees slightly bent. Press the tips of your fingers and thumbs together 6" below your bellybutton. Bend your elbows slightly. Relax your shoulders.

2

Inhale deeply as you slowly push your hands with steady force low and back to your right, then up to the height of your right shoulder. Remember to keep your *left* elbow locked in the same, slightly bent angle that you started with. Shift your weight to the ball of your right foot. Let your hands push your body into a gentle twist—don't swing. Stand tall, chin in.

3

Exhale completely as you slowly push your hands with steady force back down below your bellybutton. Keep your *left* elbow locked. With continuous motion, push your hands low and back, then on up to your left to the height of your left shoulder, now keeping your *right* elbow locked in the same, slightly bent position that you started with in Step 1. Shift your weight to the ball of your left foot. Twist only as far as comfortable. Continue back to your right and repeat.

EXTENDED OVERHEAD PULL

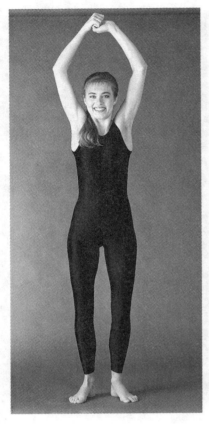 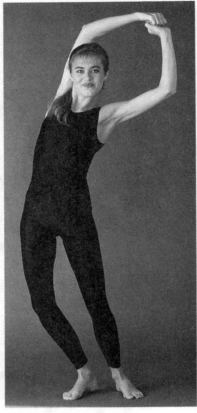 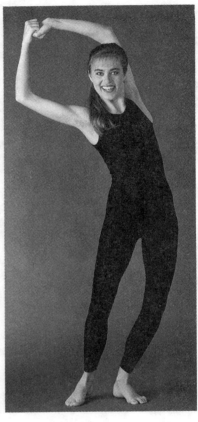

1

Stand with your heels 6" apart, feet angled out. Hook your fingers together. Extend your arms high above your head, pulled toward the rear as far as you can. Bend your elbows slightly. Stand tall, don't stick your chin out. Smile!

2

Inhale deeply as you slowly pull your hands with steady force over your right shoulder. Remember to keep your hands and elbows back and both of your elbows locked in the same, slightly bent position that you started with. Shift your weight to the ball of your left foot while keeping your knees slightly bent. Sway your hips to your left. Be sure to inhale all the way across the motion. Hold your head high and straight forward.

3

Exhale completely as you slowly pull your hands with steady force back over your head and over your left shoulder. Remember to keep your hands and elbows back and both of your elbows locked in the same, slightly bent position that you started with in Step 1. Shift your weight to the ball of your right foot. Sway your hips to your right. Be sure to exhale all the way across the motion. Continue back to your right and repeat.

EXTENDED OVERHEAD PUSH

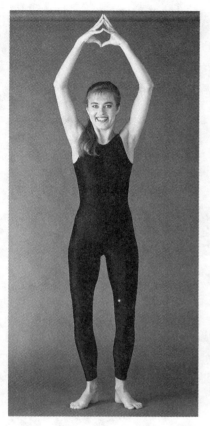 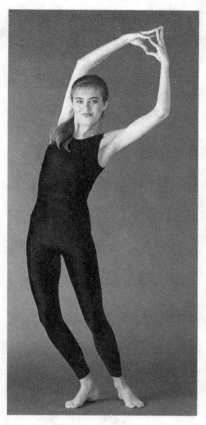 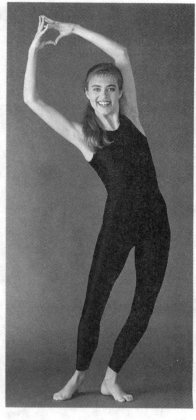

1

Stand with your heels 6" apart, feet angled out. Press the tips of your fingers and thumbs together. Extend your arms high above your head, pushed toward the rear as far as you can. Bend your elbows slightly. Smile!

2

Inhale deeply as you slowly push your hands with steady force over your right shoulder. Remember to keep your hands and elbows back and both of your elbows locked in the same, slightly bent position that you started with. Shift your weight to the ball of your left foot. Sway your hips to your left. Sway your body only as far as you can while keeping your head straight up. Stand tall, chin in.

3

Exhale completely as you slowly push your hands with steady force back over your head and over your left shoulder. Remember to keep your hands and elbows pushed back, and both of your elbows locked in the same, slightly bent position that you started with in Step 1. Shift your weight to the ball of your right foot. Sway your hips to your right. Concentrate on keeping your knees slightly bent and your hips tucked under throughout the motion. Continue back to your right and repeat.

EXTENDED BEHIND-THE-BACK PULL

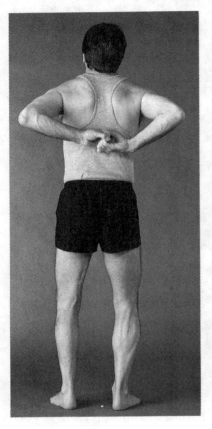 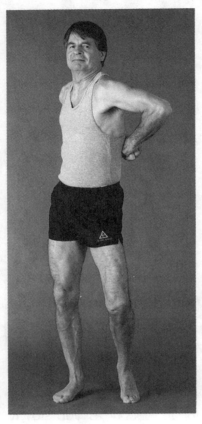 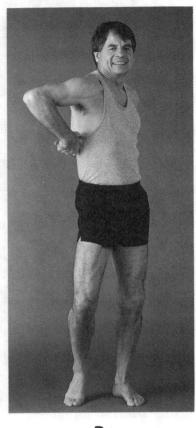

1

Stand with your heels 6" apart, feet angled out. Hook your fingers together behind your back and as high up on your spine as possible. Relax your shoulders. Smile!

2

Inhale deeply as you slowly pull your hands with steady force to your right. Pull your hands as high and as far forward as possible on your right rib cage. Point your right elbow forward for a good flex. Shift your weight to the ball of your left foot while keeping your knees slightly bent. Hold your head high and straight forward.

3

Exhale completely as you slowly pull your hands with steady force back to your left. Pull your hands as high and as far forward as possible on your left rib cage. Point your left elbow forward for a good flex. Shift your weight to the ball of your right foot. Don't put your weight on your heels. Stand tall, chin in. Continue back to your right and repeat.

EXTENDED BEHIND-THE-BACK PUSH

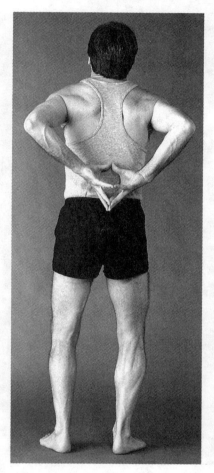

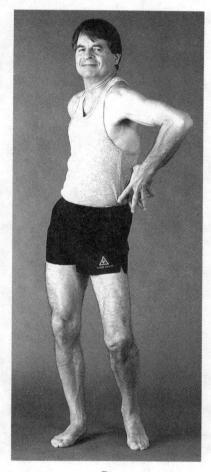

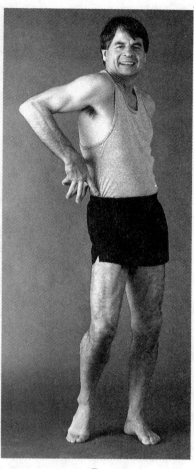

1

Stand with your heels 6" apart, feet angled out. Press the tips of your fingers and thumbs together behind your back and as high up on your spine as possible. Stand with Perfect Posture. Relax your shoulders. Smile!

2

Inhale deeply as you slowly push your hands with steady force to your right. Push your hands as high and as far forward as possible on your right rib cage. Point your right elbow forward for a good flex. Shift your weight to the ball of your left foot. Concentrate on keeping the motion smooth and fluid. Hold your head high and straight forward.

3

Exhale completely as you slowly push your hands with steady force back to your left. Push your hands as high and as far forward as possible on your left rib cage. Point your left elbow forward for a full flex. Shift your weight to the ball of your right foot. Be sure to keep your knees slightly bent with your hips tucked under. Continue back to your right and repeat.

BRAINSTORMS AND ENERGY BURSTS

YOUR PERSONAL PROGRESS RECORD

DATE	WEIGHT	WAIST	HIPS	THIGHS	CHEST	STRENGTH (1–10)
____	_____	_____	_____	_____	_____	_____

COORDINATION (1–10)	ENERGY (1–10)	RELAXED (1–10)	SLEEP (1–10)
_____	_____	_____	_____

ELIMINATION (1–10)	EATING HABITS (1–10)	FACE (1–10)	OVERALL APPEARANCE (1–10)
_____	_____	_____	_____

OVERALL FEELINGS (1–10)   NOTE: Score 1 as low and 10 as high.

_____

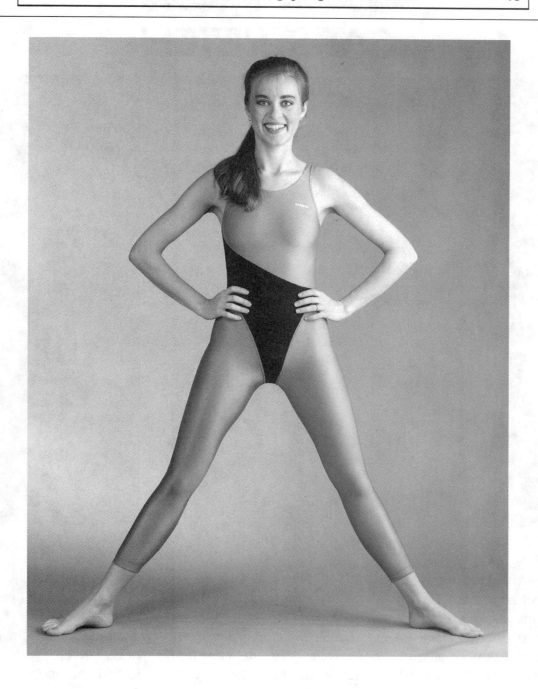

LEG SYNERGETICS

Your legs, like the rest of your body, are originals, and you can keep these wonderful limbs strong and shapely as long as you exercise them regularly. Adding Leg Synergetics to your workout can develop legs and buttocks as beautifully conditioned as a dancer's or an athlete's. Exercising your legs also helps increase your heart's ability to circulate oxygen-rich blood throughout your lower extremities.

You can combine Leg Synergetics with your Rainbows (Stepping Out Plus) or you can do them separately during your workouts, or at other times during the day. Stepping Out Plus is an even more effective no-impact aerobic exercise.

CAT STRETCH

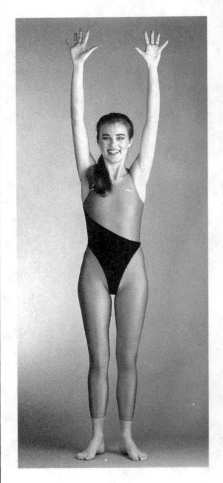
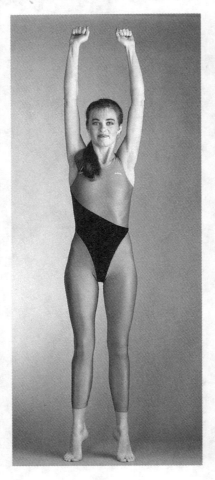
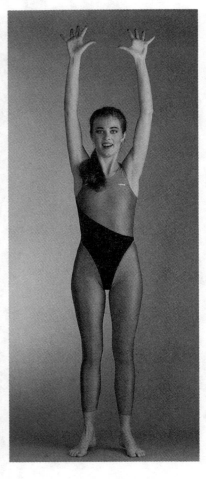

1

Stand with your heels 6" apart, feet angled out. Extend your arms straight up over your head on either side of your ears. Lock your elbows. Face your palms forward. Smile!

2

Inhale deeply as you slowly go up onto your toes as far as your ankle joints will allow. Slowly close your hands so that they are clenched tightly at the peak of your stretch. Stand tall, chin in.

3

Exhale completely as you slowly bring your heels down to just above the floor. Do not put any weight on your heels. Keep your elbows locked and open your hands. Stretch your fingers backward as hard as you can. Take two counts to go up on your toes and two counts to come down. Keep your shoulders relaxed. Repeat.

CAT STRETCH: VARIATIONS
4 VARIATIONS

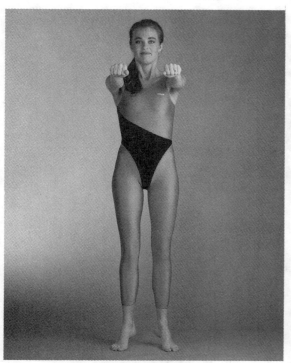

Arms extended out front

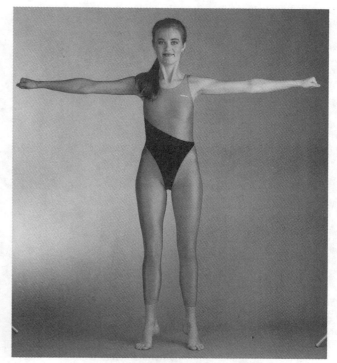

Arms extended out to side

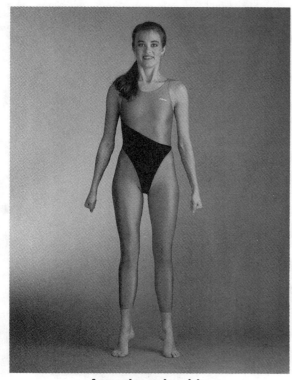

Arms down by side

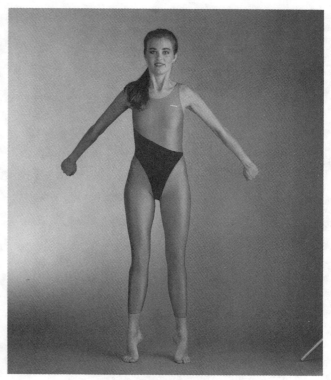

Arms behind back

CAT STRETCH
4 HAND POSITIONS
(Use all four hand positions with all four variations.)

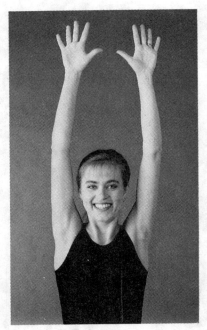

palms forward

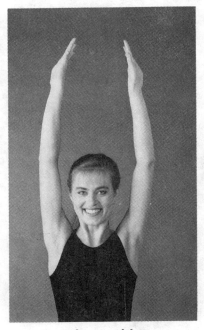

palms to side

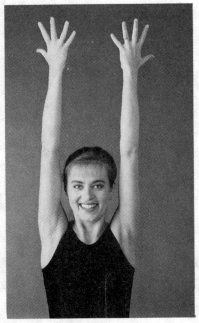

palms to back

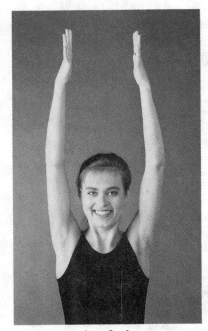

palms facing

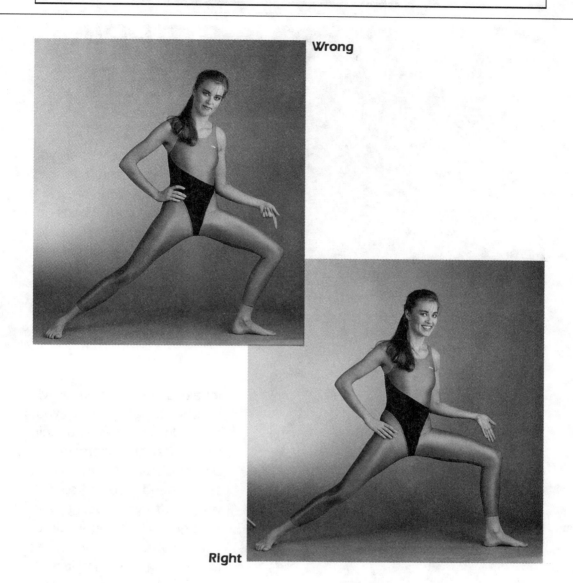

Wrong

Right

STEPPING OUT THE RIGHT WAY

Your knee joints are designed to carry your natural weight upright. They are not designed to be overloaded with excessive body weight or awkward positions. Since your joints must last a lifetime, they must be treated with gentleness and care.

To minimize joint degeneration, avoid deep knee bends, hard dancing, excessive jogging, jumping, or anything that exerts undue stress on your back, hips, knees, ankles, and other joints.

The left photograph demonstrates the wrong and stressful way to perform the Stepping Out, which places undue strain on your knee joint. If your knee is pushed too far forward, it can be stressed.

The photograph on the right shows you the correct, safe, and effective way to do a Stepping Out. Spread your legs so that it is all you can do to bring your shin to an imaginary line perpendicular to the floor. This extension will give your legs and behind a good stretch to keep them firm and fit.

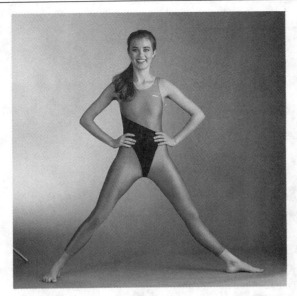

STEPPING OUT

1

Spread your feet until you feel your inside thigh muscles tighten. Point your toes forward. Place your hands on your hips. Turn your right foot out to your right. Balance yourself comfortably or hold onto something for support until your balance improves. Smile!

2

Inhale deeply as you slowly bend your right knee to your right. Do not allow your shin to go past an imaginary line perpendicular to the floor. Don't bend your torso forward. (If you don't feel enough pull on the inside of your thighs, spread your feet further apart so that it is all you can do to bring your shin to the perpendicular.)

3

Exhale completely as you slowly straighten your leg. Gently lock your knee and then repeat. Do this in a steady rhythm of two counts down, two counts back. Do repetitions to the left by switching legs. Hold your head high and straight forward.

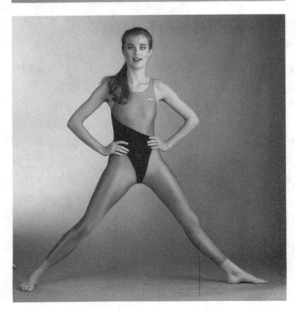

STEPPING OUT PLUS (CHEST-HIGH PULL)

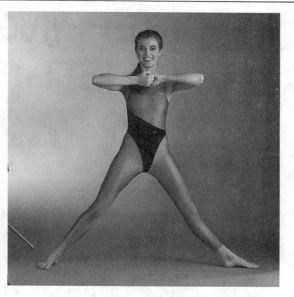

1

Spread your feet until you feel your inside thigh muscles tighten. Point your toes forward. Hook your fingers. Hold your hands and elbows at shoulder level with your elbows bent at right angles. Turn your right foot out to your right. Balance yourself comfortably. Smile!

2

Inhale deeply as you slowly bend your right knee to your right. Pull your hands with steady force to your right as far as you can. Hold your arms at shoulder level and keep your left elbow locked at a right angle. Do not allow your shin to go past an imaginary line perpendicular to the floor. Don't lean forward.

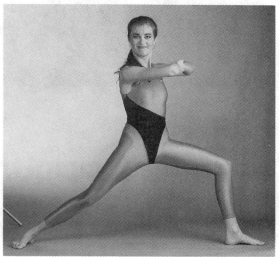

3

Exhale completely as you slowly straighten your knee, feeling a stretch, and pull your hands back to the center of your chest. Hold your elbows at shoulder level. Make this motion a steady rhythm of two counts down, two counts back. Do to the left by switching legs. Hold your head high and straight forward.

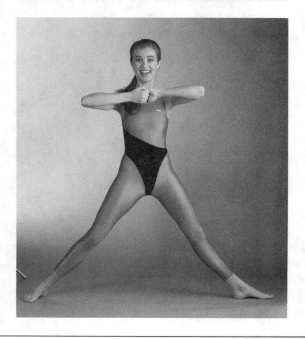

STEPPING OUT PLUS CHEST-HIGH PUSH

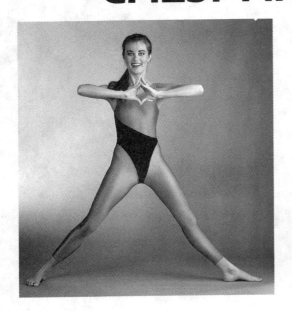 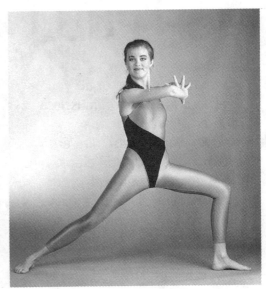

STEPPING OUT PLUS OVERHEAD PULL

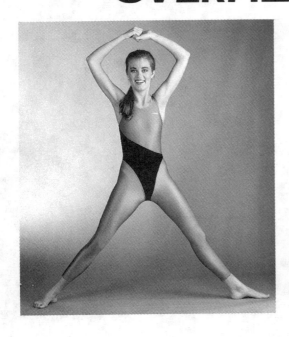 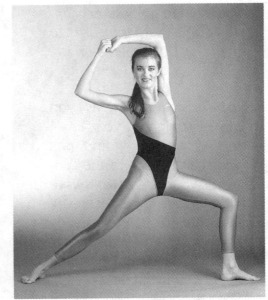

STEPPING OUT PLUS LOW PUSH

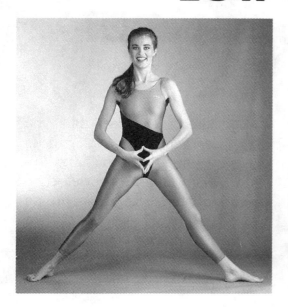 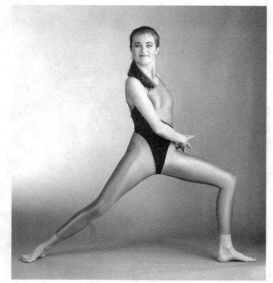

STEPPING OUT PLUS BEHIND-THE-BACK PULL

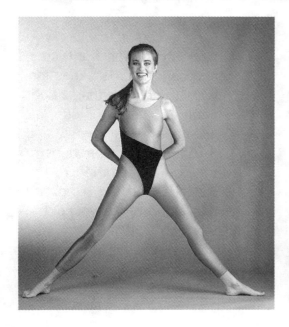 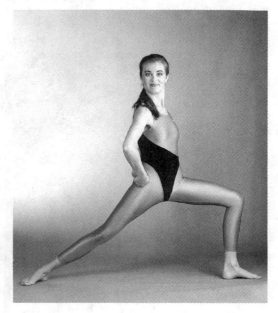

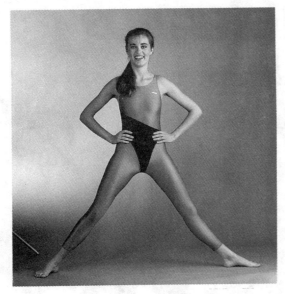

DOUBLE STEPPING OUT

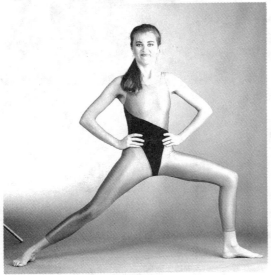

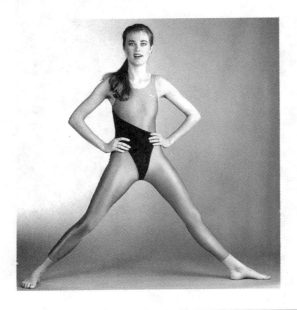

1

Spread your feet until you feel your inside thigh muscles tighten. Point your toes forward. Balance yourself comfortably. Place your hands on your hips. Turn your right foot out to your right. This exercise is not for anybody with weak knees. Smile!

2

Inhale deeply as you bend your right knee to your right. Do not allow your shin to go past an imaginary line perpendicular to the floor.

3

Exhale completely as you straighten your right knee and bend your left knee forward to no more than a right angle. Straighten your left knee and repeat steps 2 and 3. After doing repetitions to the right, do to the left. You can also add the hand and arm motions like you did in Stepping Out Plus.

STEPPING OUT HEEL LIFT

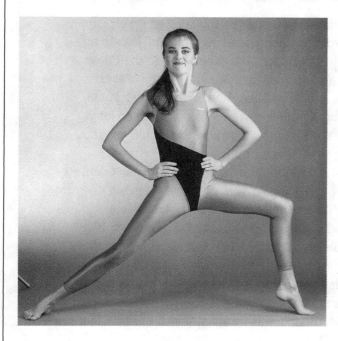

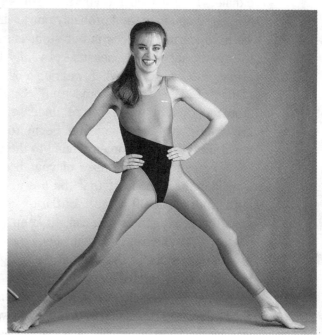

When doing the Stepping Out, lift the heel of the "bending" leg off of the floor throughout the entire bending and straightening. When you straighten your leg, point your toe and really stretch your calf and thigh muscle. Smile!

POWER BREATHING REVIEW

How are you progressing with your breathing? Have you got the hang of it yet? For most people it takes quite a while to reprogram their breathing pattern. Breathing with your diaphragm is probably a new body motion for you. When you do the Power Breathing along with the rest of the body motions, you've got a lot to think about!

Refer to the earlier Power Breathing section if you like. Practice inhaling through your nose as you expand your stomach muscles, filling your lower and upper lungs with air. Exhale from your open, relaxed mouth with an audible "aaaahhh" as you contract your stomach muscles, squeezing all the old air out.

You may be asking yourself, "Why should I breathe this way? It doesn't feel natural to expand my stomach muscles on the inhale and contract them on the exhale. My body wants to do the opposite!" Remember, you are now finally learning how to breathe correctly. Watch babies and young children breathing. They breathe by expanding their stomachs on the inhale and letting their stomachs fall on the exhale. Take a look for yourself. All warm-blooded creatures breathe this way—horses, dogs, cats, and probably our prehistoric ancestors. Somehow in our culture, we have learned to suck in our stomachs in an unnatural way. We may have learned to breathe incorrectly because of vanity (you don't want your stomach sticking out every time you inhale when wearing a bikini!). Or it may have come from the military stance of "Chest out, stomach in!" Or it could be from stress. You can feel your stomach tighten when you're under stress, can't you? Children watch how the grown-ups are breathing and begin to copy that same breathing habit and so, unnatural breathing comes around to the next generation again, full circle.

Oxygen is *the life force* of your body. Without it you would very quickly die. Consider for a moment that the average human brain weighs three pounds, yet it burns more than 30 percent of the oxygen we breathe in. You must be sure to take in as much oxygen as you can, to keep your mind sharp and working clearly and to ensure that the rest of your body gets its fair share of oxygen too. Improper breathing results in the premature aging of the body. Your body cells age quickly from hypoxia—lack of oxygen.

Start by consciously Power Breathing with every Synergetics motion you do. Every day. You can also practice your Power Breathing while you are driving to work, watching TV, at a movie, at a desk, in the kitchen—anywhere you are. Do your Fantastic Faces at the same time! This natural way of breathing will begin to rejuvenate your body, increase your energy, and help keep you from prematurely aging.

CUSTOMIZING SYNERGETICS

It's fun to make up your own custom workout programs. You know what your body needs, so why not take charge and give it what's best for you. With a couple of simple formulas, you can quickly figure out how many of each exercise makes up a total of 12 minutes, 24 minutes, 3 minutes, whatever length workout you want. Just remember these important facts:

- There are 720 seconds in a 12-minute workout. There are 86,400 seconds or 1,440 minutes in every day. You have plenty of time for Synergetics.

- Each Rainbow repetition (a right to left motion) takes about 4 seconds if you exercise at the Basic Tempo. This means that you can do 180 repetitions (right to left) in a 12-minute workout.

- There are 8 basic hand positions in the Basic Rainbows and 8 basic hand positions in the Extended Rainbows. This means that if you wanted to do 10 of each of the Basic Rainbows, you would be doing 80 repetitions, or a little less than half of your 12-minute workout. If you wanted to do 10 each of the Extended Rainbows and 10 each of the Basic Rainbows, you would be doing 160 repetitions. This leaves 20 repetitions that you could do with Leg Synergetics, for instance, which will fill up your 12-minute workout.

- The secret to a versatile body is to develop a versatile series of workout programs. Keep your body guessing as to what motions you are going to ask it to do in your next workout. You don't want your body to become bored, because that means that your mind will become bored, and if that happens, then you are just going through the motions and might as well go back to bed.

Here's a summary of the Synergetics exercises you have learned so far. You can refer to this list when you are customizing your workouts.

BASIC RAINBOWS	EXTENDED RAINBOWS
Chest-High Pull	Extended Chest-High Pull
Chest-High Push	Extended Chest-High Push
Low Pull	Extended Low Pull
Low Push	Extended Low Push
Overhead Pull	Extended Overhead Pull
Overhead Push	Extended Overhead Push
Behind-the-Back Pull	Extended Behind-the-Back Pull
Behind-the-Back Push	Extended Behind-the-Back Push

FANTASTIC FACES	LEG SYNERGETICS
The Hunter	Cat Stretch
The Popeye	Cat Stretch Variations
The Guppy	Stepping Out
The Gorilla	Stepping Out Plus
	Double Stepping Out
	Stepping Out Heel Lift

POWER BREATHING

Below are some blanks for you to fill for your customized workouts. Decide when and where you want to work out. Because Synergetics can be done almost anywhere, you can come up with some pretty imaginative times and places to take a Synergetics break. Here is a sample workout and some blank space for you to create your own daily programs for the coming weeks. Include your Power Breathing and Fantastic Faces!

CUSTOM WORKOUT ONE

Total Time: _12 Minutes_

Place: _at home_

Time of Day: _before breakfast_

Do in sequence:

10 of each **Basic** Rainbow

5 of each **Extended** Rainbow

20 Stepping Out Plus

20 Cat Stretch Variations

Fantastic Face: The Hunter

CUSTOM WORKOUT TWO

Total Time: _12 Minutes_

Place: _____

Time of Day: _____

Do in sequence:

_____

_____

_____

_____

Fantastic Face: _____

CUSTOM WORKOUT THREE

Total Time: _12 Minutes_

Place: _____

Time of Day: _____

Do in sequence:

_____

_____

_____

_____

Fantastic Face: _____

CUSTOM WORKOUT FOUR

Total Time: _12 Minutes_

Place: _____

Time of Day: _____

Do in sequence:

_____

_____

_____

_____

Fantastic Face: _____

CUSTOM WORKOUT FIVE

Total Time: 12 Minutes

Place: _____

Time of Day: _____

Do in sequence:

_____

_____

_____

_____

Fantastic Face: _____

CUSTOM WORKOUT SIX

Total Time: 12 Minutes

Place: _____

Time of Day: _____

Do in sequence:

_____

_____

_____

_____

Fantastic Face: _____

CUSTOM WORKOUT SEVEN

Total Time: 12 Minutes

Place: _____

Time of Day: _____

Do in sequence:

_____

_____

_____

_____

Fantastic Face: _____

CUSTOM WORKOUT EIGHT

Total Time: 12 Minutes

Place: _____

Time of Day: _____

Do in sequence:

_____

_____

_____

_____

Fantastic Face: _____

PERFECT FORM CHECKLIST

You can't check your form often enough. Learn the right moves now and you will have them for life.

	CHECK ONE	
	YES	**NO**
Are you smiling?	_____	_____
Are you holding your head high and facing forward?	_____	_____
Are you Power Breathing—expanding and contracting your stomach muscles?	_____	_____
Are you doing a Fantastic Face?	_____	_____
Are you keeping your chin tucked?	_____	_____
Are you pulling and pushing with constant force and speed?	_____	_____
Are you developing a smooth, consistent rhythm?	_____	_____
Are you holding your hands and elbows at the correct level?	_____	_____
Are you coming to a gentle stop without jerking?	_____	_____
Are you holding your elbows locked at the instructed angle?	_____	_____
Are you pulling and pushing with enough resistance?	_____	_____
Are you giving yourself enough time to inhale and exhale as deeply and completely as possible?	_____	_____
Are you pulling and pushing your body to the maximum without ducking or turning your head?	_____	_____
Are you keeping your hips tucked under your shoulders?	_____	_____
Are you keeping your weight from collapsing on your hips?	_____	_____
Are you gently twisting your body without swaying your hips?	_____	_____
Are you shifting your weight to the proper foot?	_____	_____

Are you keeping your knees slightly bent? _____ _____

Are you keeping your heels 6" apart, toes turned
outward? _____ _____

Are you shifting your weight completely from one foot to
the other? _____ _____

SYNERGETICS FEELINGS

By now you've seen many changes and felt many positive feelings. The more
conscious you are of your positive feelings, the more you will enjoy them. Let's run
down the list of positive Synergetics Feelings.

	CHECK ONE	
	YES	**NO**

Do you feel your spine and neck pleasantly flexing as you
pull or push into a sway or a twist? _____ _____

Do you feel your thigh, calf, and buttock muscles tighten
on the side where you shift your weight? _____ _____

Do you feel that you are breathing more deeply? _____ _____

Do you feel energized after your Synergetics workouts? _____ _____

Do you feel growing sensations in your muscle fibers? _____ _____

Do you feel your heart rate increase as you work out? _____ _____

Do you feel stronger? _____ _____

Do you feel more calm after a set of Synergetics? _____ _____

Do you feel that you are standing up straighter and
walking taller? _____ _____

Do you feel that you are sleeping better? _____ _____

Do you feel yourself getting more grace and balance? _____ _____

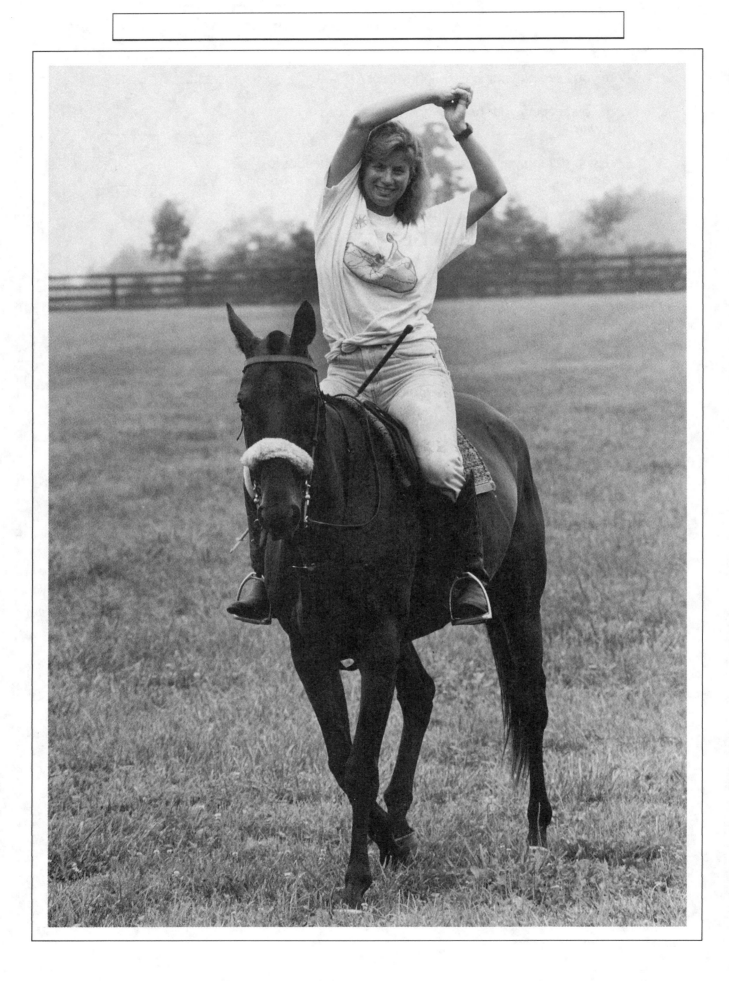

6

Hand Synergetics

The Rainbow Series and the Leg Synergetics can keep your body in exceptional shape, but it is important to add some variations to your daily programs which focus on new sets of muscles and body coordination.

The first group of supplemental exercises is Hand Synergetics. You can add one or several of them to your workouts as you choose. They are an enjoyable way to condition your entire body with increased focus on your hands. They can help you increase your hand strength, circulation, and flexibility.

Our hands got a good workout in the days when we had to spin, weave, knit, churn, scrub, hoe, plow, chop, and weed. But just like hunting and gathering, vigorous hand work for most people is almost a thing of the past. Because we live in a push-button society, our hands don't get enough exercise and become weak and fragile way before their natural time.

Your hands must get a good amount of exercise every day if you want to keep them from withering and becoming arthritic. If your hands are not functional, then it is difficult for you to take care of the rest of your body.

Continue doing your Fantastic Faces with these Hand Synergetics. The Guppy goes well with The Hook and its variations.

THE ROOSTER (BASIC)

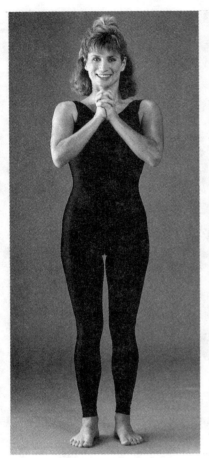 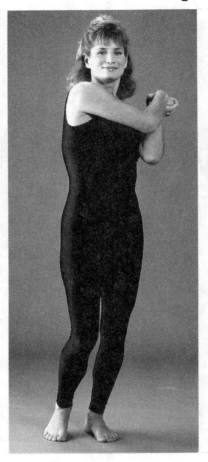 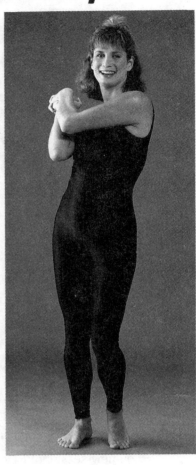

1

Stand with your heels 6" apart, feet angled out. Remember to keep your weight on the balls of your feet. Clasp your hands by interlacing your fingers. Hold them close to your chin. Point your elbows down with your knuckles up. Smile!

2

Inhale deeply as you push your hands with steady force to your right. Bend your resisting right hand back at the wrist with your left hand. Shift your weight to the ball of your right foot. Gently push your body into a tight right twist. Hold your head high and straight forward.

3

Exhale completely as you push your hands with steady force back to your left. Bend your resisting left hand back at the wrist with your right hand. Shift your weight to the ball of your left foot. Gently push your body into a tight left twist. Keep your knees slightly bent and your hips tucked under.

THE HOOK (CHEST-HIGH)

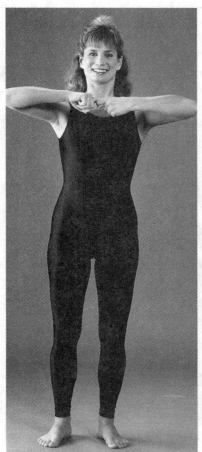

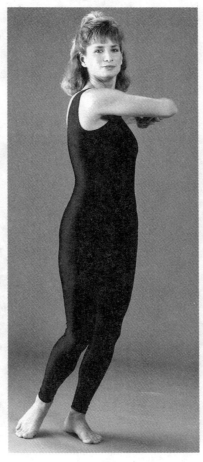

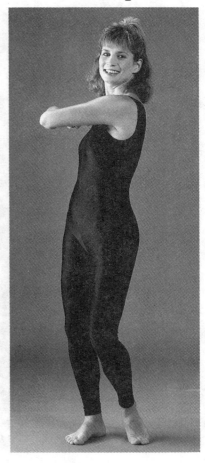

1

Stand with your heels 6" apart, feet angled out. Hook just your index fingers 8" from your chest. Hold your hands and elbows at shoulder level. Smile!

2

Inhale deeply as you pull your hands with steady force to your right. Remember to hold your arms at shoulder level. Shift your weight to the ball of your right foot while keeping your knees slightly bent. Hold your head high and straight forward.

3

Exhale completely as you pull your hands with steady force to your left. Remember to hold your arms at shoulder level. Shift your weight to the ball of your left foot. Hold your head high, chin in. Continue back to your right and repeat.

THE ROOSTER (VARIATIONS)

You can use the Rainbow arm positions with the Rooster hand position. The body form is identical to the form in the Rainbow Series; only the hand position is different. You can do the Rooster with hands clasped or with your fingertips pushing.

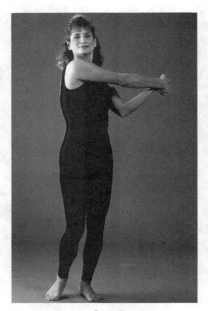

Arms Out Front

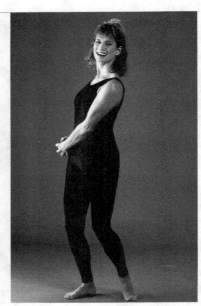

Arms Low

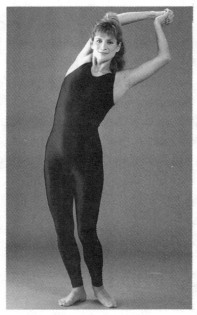

Arms Overhead

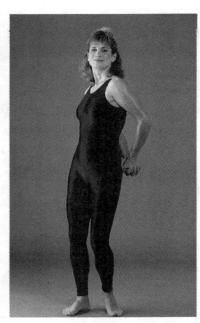

Arms Behind Back

THE HOOK (VARIATIONS)

The Hook also uses the identical body motions of the Basic and Extended Rainbows.

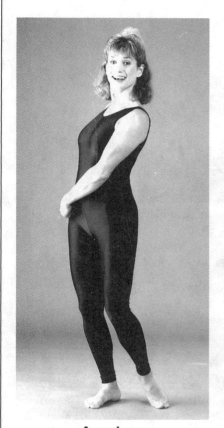

Arms Low

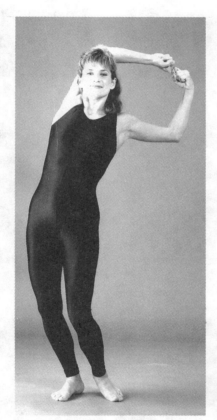

Arms Overhead

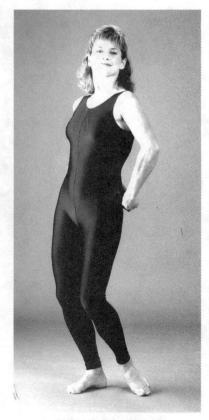

Arms Behind Back

THE HOOK (FINGER GRIPS)

Every time you change the position of your hands and hook your different fingers, you are educating your body to coordinate new combinations of muscles to perform the motion.

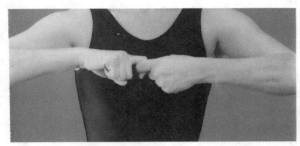

Index Finger

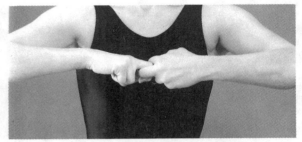

Second Finger

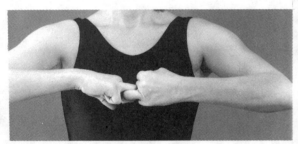

Ring Finger

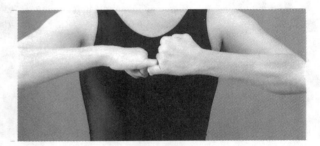

Little Finger

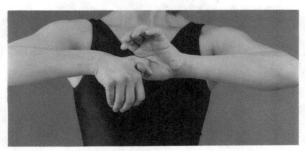

Thumb

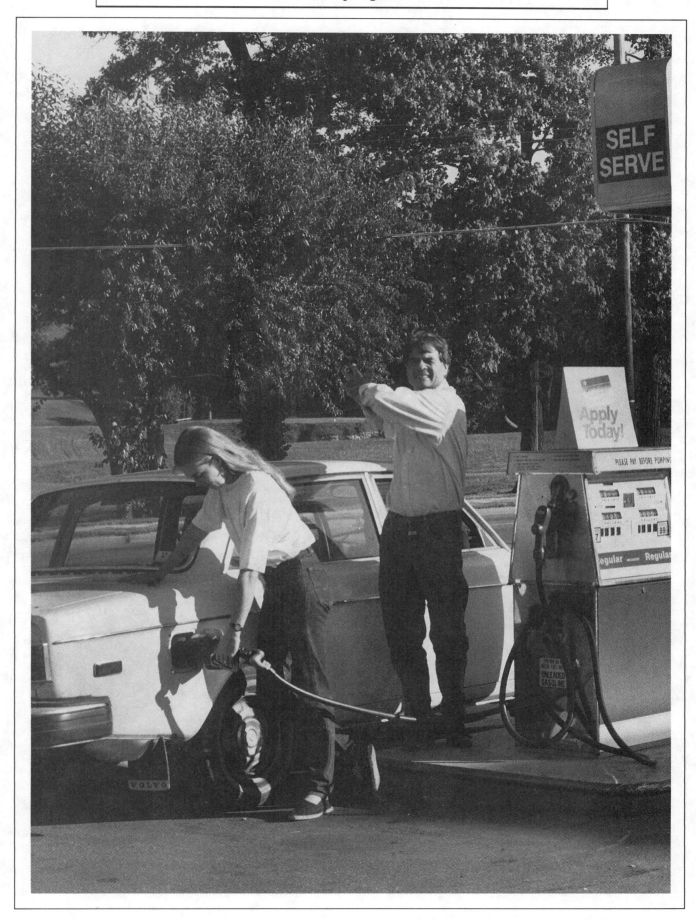

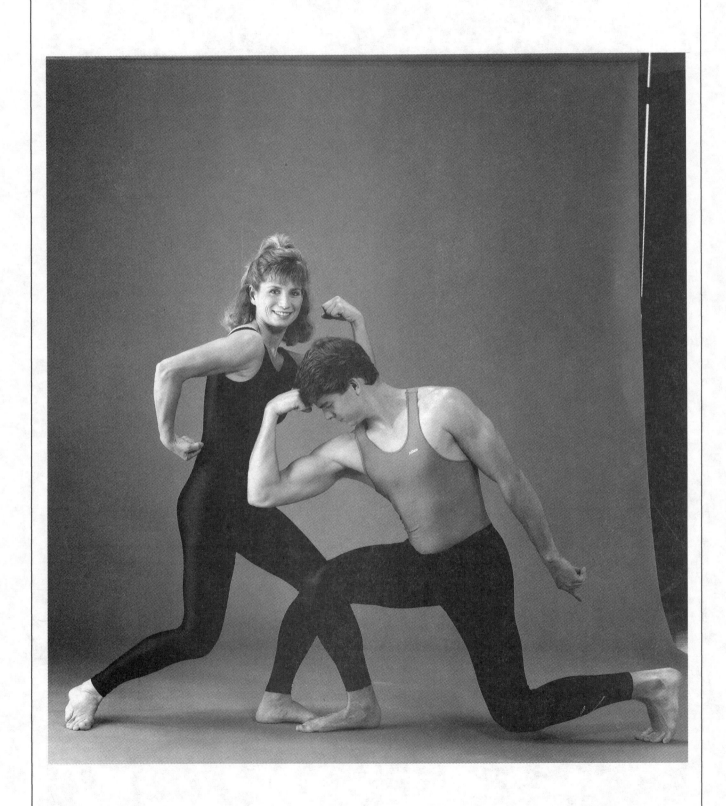

7

Power Synergetics

The word *power* can mean a lot of different things. You don't have to hold up the world like Atlas did, or bench-press three hundred pounds, but wouldn't it be nice to have some extra power in reserve—just in case?

Power Synergetics are for everybody. The difference between these exercises and the Rainbows, for example, is that the hands and arms are positioned in such a way that you can pull or push with even more force if you want to. Power Synergetics also hook together entirely different muscle combinations which can develop even more strength, coordination, and muscle separation in your body. You can use Power Synergetics as a relaxing change of pace and posture for your body, or you can bear down and get an endurance workout that will challenge even a professional athlete.

You'll like doing the Gorilla Fantastic Face with Pumping The Well since your arm action allows you to stretch your face and neck to their maximum. Choose the Fantastic Faces you like best with the rest of the Power Synergetics.

PUMPING THE WELL

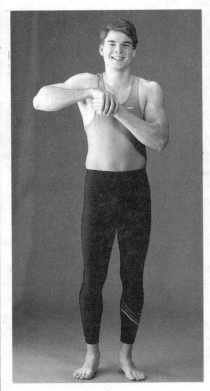

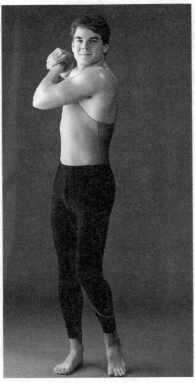

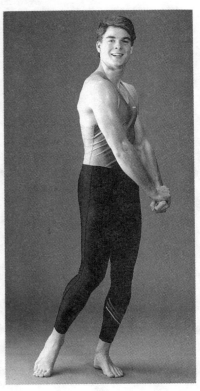

1

Stand with your heels 6" apart, feet angled out. Make your right hand into a loosely closed fist and place it, palm in, against the left side of your chest. Place your left hand on top of your right fist with your fingers pointing down on the back of your fist and your thumb on the inside of your fist. Point your right elbow down and keep your left elbow at shoulder height. Smile!

2

Inhale deeply as you lift your hands up to near your left ear. Point your left elbow up. Do this without resistance. Shift your weight to the ball of your left foot while keeping your knees slightly bent.

3

Exhale completely as you push your hands with steady force down across your body until both elbows gently lock with your hands at your right hip. Shift your weight to the ball of your right foot. Take your hands back up to your left ear without resistance, shift your weight back to your left and repeat steps 2 and 3. Do equal repetitions with the other hand. Try Pumping The Well with your knuckles pointing down and with your knuckles pointing up for new muscle combinations. You can also make this a pull motion by having your left hand pull up on your right hand as your right hand pulls down to your hip.

STEPPING OUT WITH PUMPING THE WELL

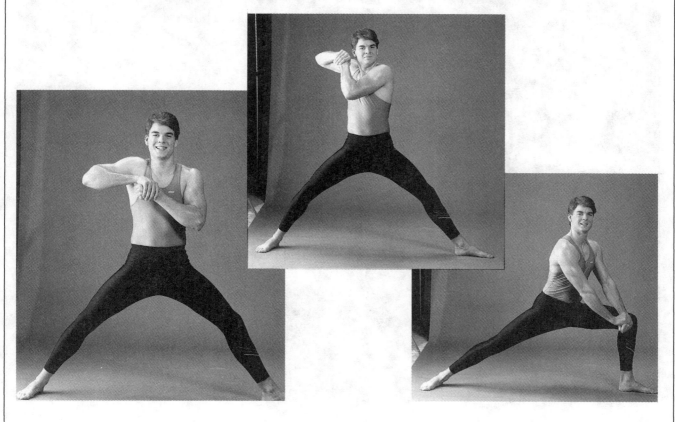

1

Spread your feet until you feel your inside thigh muscles tighten. Balance yourself comfortably. Make your right hand into a loosely closed fist and place it, palm in, against the left side of your chest. Place your left hand on top of your right fist with your fingers pointing down on the back of your fist and your thumb on the inside of your fist. Point your right elbow down and keep your left elbow at shoulder height. Turn your right foot out to your right. Smile!

2

Inhale deeply as you lift your hands up to near your left ear. Point your left elbow up. Do this without resistance. Don't allow your body to tilt forward. Hold your head high.

3

Exhale completely as you push your hands with steady force down across your body until both elbows gently lock with your hands at your right knee. Bend your right knee to your right. Do not allow your shin to go past an imaginary line perpendicular to the floor. On the inhale, straighten your leg and let your hands float back up to your left ear without resistance and repeat. Do equal repetitions with the other hand and leg.

ARM WRESTLE

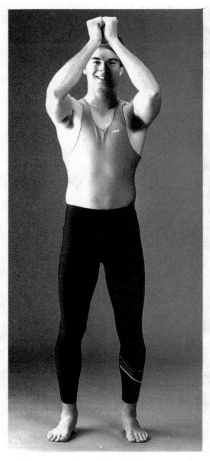 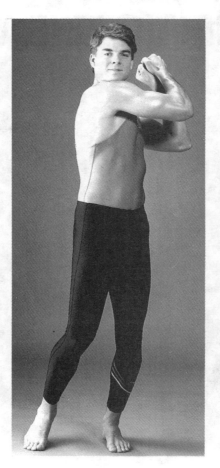 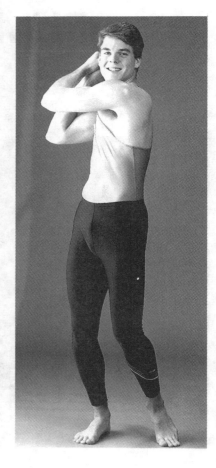

1

Stand with your heels 6″ apart, feet angled out and your knees slightly bent. Press your fists together (palms facing each other) in front of your forehead. Hold your elbows at shoulder level with your knuckles pointing up. You can really use a lot of force on this exercise. Smile!

2

Inhale deeply as you push your fists with steady force to your right and down beside your right ear. Twist your wrists so that your left fist is on top. Bend your resisting right fist back with your pushing left fist. Hold your elbows at shoulder level. Shift your weight to the ball of your right foot. Hold your head high and straight forward.

3

Exhale completely as you push your fists with steady force back across to your left and down beside your left ear. Twist your wrists so that your right fist is on top. Bend your resisting left fist back with your pushing right fist. Hold your elbows at shoulder level. Shift your weight to the ball of your left foot. Hold your head high and straight with your chin in. Continue back to your right and repeat.

BRAINSTORMS AND ENERGY BURSTS

YOUR PERSONAL PROGRESS RECORD

DATE	WEIGHT	WAIST	HIPS	THIGHS	CHEST	STRENGTH (1–10)

COORDINATION (1–10)	ENERGY (1–10)	RELAXED (1–10)	SLEEP (1–10)

ELIMINATION (1–10)	EATING HABITS (1–10)	FACE (1–10)	OVERALL APPEARANCE (1–10)

OVERALL FEELINGS (1–10)   NOTE: Score 1 as low and 10 as high.

AROUND-THE-WORLD PULL

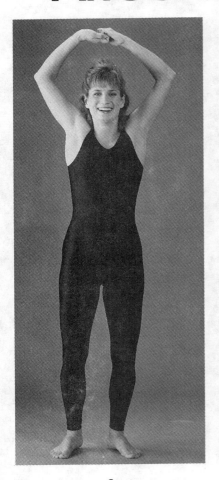
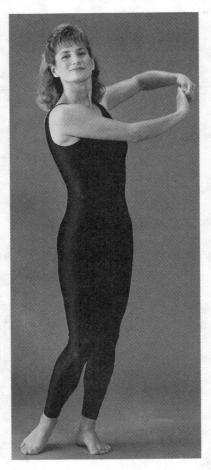
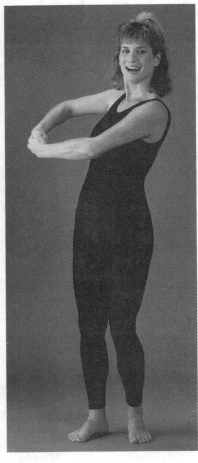

1

Stand with your heels 6" apart, feet angled out. Hook your fingers 3" over your head. Pull your hands and elbows toward the rear. Smile!

2

Inhale deeply as you pull your hands with steady force out and down to your right in a clockwise, circular motion. Shift your weight to the ball of your right foot while keeping your knees slightly bent. Pull your hands close to your body and 6" below your bellybutton. Stand tall, chin in.

3

Exhale completely as you continue the circular motion by pulling your hands with steady force up and out to your left. Shift your weight to the ball of your left foot. Pull your hands in a clockwise motion back over your head. Continue the circular motion as you do more repetitions. This exercise should also be done counterclockwise.

AROUND-THE-WORLD PUSH

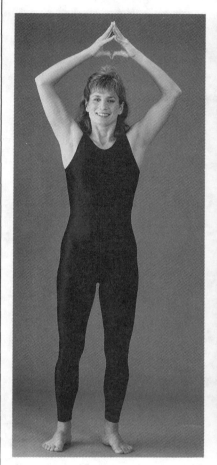

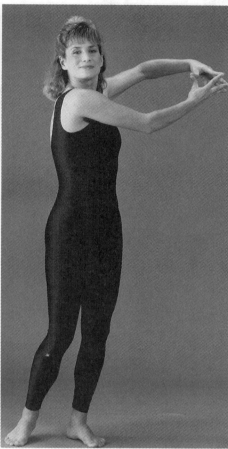

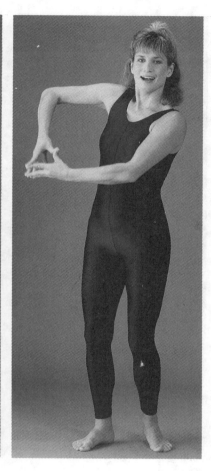

1

Stand with your heels 6" apart, feet angled out and your knees slightly bent. Press the tips of your fingers and thumbs together 3" over your head. Push your hands and elbows toward the rear. Smile!

2

Inhale deeply as you push your hands with steady force out and down to your right in a clockwise, circular motion. Shift your weight to the ball of your right foot. Push your hands close to your body and 6" below your bellybutton.

3

Exhale completely as you continue the circular motion by pushing your hands with steady force up and out to your left. Shift your weight to the ball of your left foot. Push your hands in a clockwise motion to back over your head. Continue the circular motion as you do more repetitions. This exercise should also be done counterclockwise. Hold your head high and straight forward.

PADDLING PULL

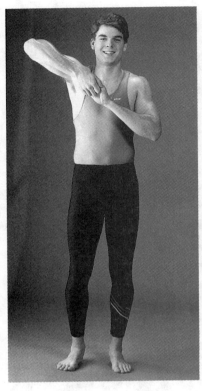

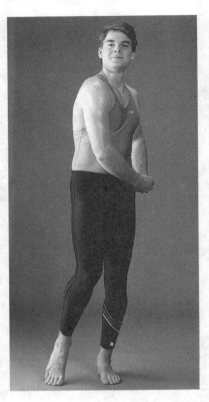

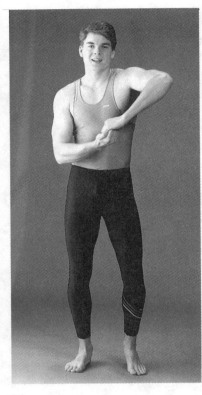

1

Stand with your heels 6″ apart, feet angled out and your knees slightly bent. Hook your fingers about 8″ from your chest. Point your left elbow up over your left shoulder and point your right elbow down. Smile!

2

Inhale deeply as you pull your hands with steady force down across your body to brush your right hip. Shift your weight to the ball of your right foot. As your hands brush by your right hip, pull them low and toward the rear, then up to your right. Lead with your right elbow until it is pointing up over your right shoulder. Your left elbow is pointing down.

3

Exhale completely as you pull your hands with steady force back down and across your body to brush your left hip. Shift your weight to the ball of your left foot. As your hands brush by your left hip, pull them low and toward the rear, then up to your left. Lead with your left elbow until it is pointing up and over your left shoulder. Your right elbow is pointing down. Continue back to your right and repeat. Make the Paddling Pull one fluid, graceful motion. This exercise can also be done pulling with an upward motion instead of with a downward motion.

PADDLING PUSH

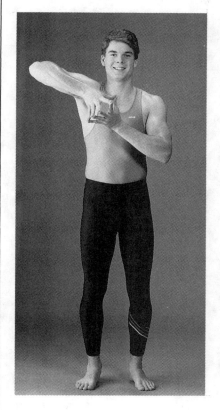

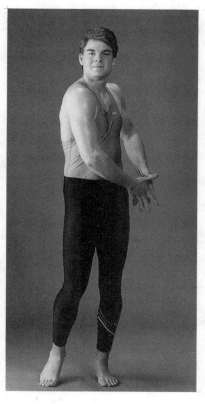

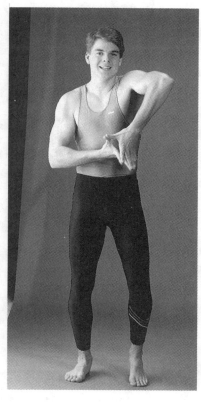

1

Stand with your heels 6″ apart, feet angled out and your knees slightly bent. Press the tips of your fingers and thumbs together about 8″ from your chest. Point your left elbow up over your left shoulder and point your right elbow down. Smile!

2

Inhale deeply as you push your hands with steady force down and across your body to brush your right hip. Shift your weight to the ball of your right foot. As your hands brush by your right hip, push them low and toward the rear, then up to the right. Lead with your right elbow until it is pointing up over your right shoulder. Your left elbow is pointing down.

3

Exhale completely as you push your hands with steady force back down and across your body to brush your left hip. Shift your weight to the ball of your left foot. As your hands brush by your left hip, push them low and toward the rear, then up to the left. Lead with your left elbow until it is pointing up and over your left shoulder. Your right elbow is pointing down. Continue back to your right and repeat. Make the Paddling Push one fluid, graceful motion. This exercise can also be done pushing with an upward motion instead of with a downward motion.

PADDLING LOW PULL

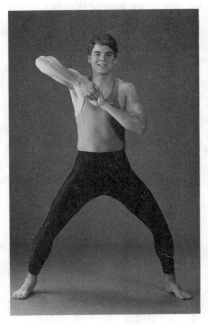

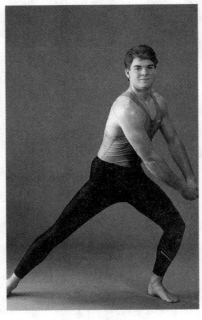

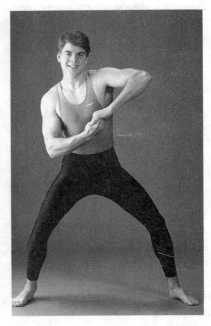

1

Stand with your heels 30" to 36" apart (depending on your height), feet angled out. Hook your fingers about 8" from your chest. Point your left elbow up over your left shoulder and point your right elbow down. Bend your knees slightly. Smile!

2

Inhale deeply as you pull your hands with steady force down across your body to brush your right knee. Shift all of your weight to your right by centering your body over your right foot and bending your right knee. Your torso does not bend or twist. Keep your back straight and your head high. As your hands brush by your right knee, pull them toward the rear. Pull your resisting hands up to your right. Lead with your right elbow until it is pointing up over your right shoulder. Your left elbow is pointing down.

3

Exhale completely as you pull your hands down and across your body to brush your left knee. Shift all of your weight to your left by centering your body over your left foot and bending your left knee. Keep your back straight and your head high. As your hands brush by your left knee, pull them toward the rear. Pull your resisting hands up to your left. Lead with your left elbow until it is pointing up over your left shoulder. Your right elbow is pointing down. Continue back to your right and repeat. Make the Paddling Low Pull one fluid, graceful motion. This exercise can also be done pulling with an upward motion instead of with a downward motion.

PADDLING LOW PUSH

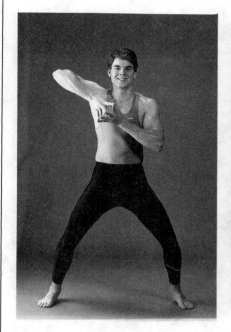

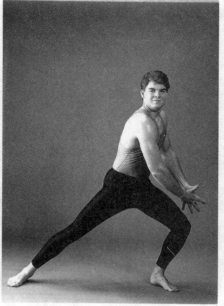

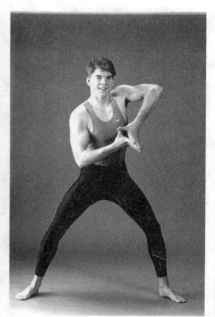

1

Stand with your heels 30" to 36" apart (depending on your height), feet angled out. Press the tips of your fingers and thumbs together about 8" from your chest. Point your left elbow up over your left shoulder and point your right elbow down. Bend your knees slightly. Smile!

2

Inhale deeply as you push your hands with steady force down across your body to brush your right knee. Shift all of your weight to your right by centering your body over your right foot and bending your right knee. Keep your back straight and your head high. As your hands brush by your right knee, push them toward the rear. Push your resisting hands up to your right. Lead with your right elbow until it is pointing up over your right shoulder. Your left elbow is pointing down.

3

Exhale deeply as you push your hands with steady force back down and across your body to brush your left knee. Shift all of your weight to your left by centering your body over your left foot and bending your left knee. Keep your back straight and your head high. As your hands brush by your left knee, push them toward the rear. Push your resisting hands up to your left. Lead with your left elbow until it is pointing up over your left shoulder. Your right elbow is pointing down. Continue back to your right and repeat. Make the Paddling Low Push one fluid, graceful motion. This exercise can also be done pushing with an upward motion instead of with a downward motion.

CHOPPING WOOD PULL

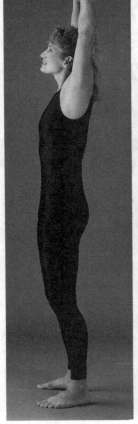
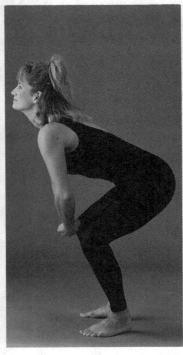
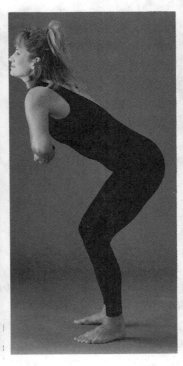
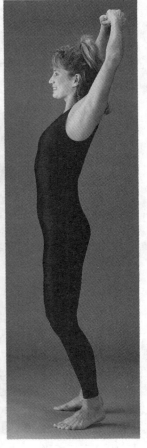

1

Stand with your heels 2' apart, feet angled out. Hook your fingers 3" over your head with your hands and elbows pulled toward your rear. Lock your elbows at right angles.

2

Inhale deeply as you slowly pull your hands with steady force out and down between your knees. Keep your elbows locked. Bend your knees at right angles. Keep your spine straight, your behind pushed back, and your head up.

3

Still inhaling, straighten your knees slightly and pull your hands up to the height of your bellybutton.

4

Exhale slowly as you bend your knees again, pulling your hands back down between your knees. Keeping your elbows locked, pull your hands out and up in front of your body and then over and as far to the rear of your head as possible. Complete your exhale as your hands come over your head. Straighten your knees to a slightly bent angle. Thrust your hips forward with your weight on the balls of both feet. Gently arch your back. Repeat Steps 2 through 4.

CHOPPING WOOD PUSH

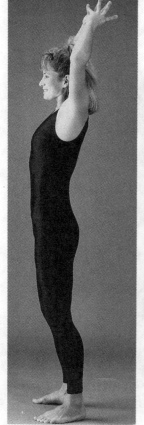

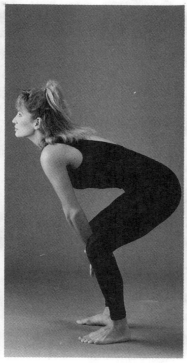

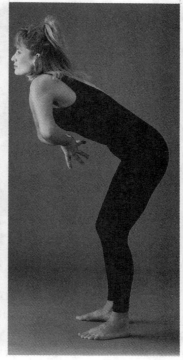

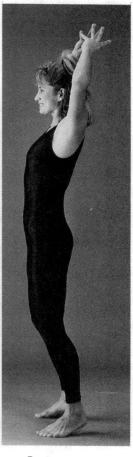

1

Stand with your heels 2' apart, feet angled out. Press the tips of your fingers and thumbs together 3" over your head with your hands and elbows pushed toward your rear. Lock your elbows at right angles. Smile!

2

Inhale deeply as you slowly push your hands with steady force out and down between your knees. Keep your elbows locked. Bend your knees at right angles. Keep your spine straight, your behind pushed back, and your head up.

3

Still inhaling, straighten your knees slightly and push your hands up to the height of your bellybutton.

4

Exhale slowly as you bend your knees again, pushing your hands back down between your knees. Keeping your elbows locked, push your hands out and up in front of your body and then over and as far to the rear of your head as possible. Complete your exhale as your hands come over your head. Straighten your knees to a slightly bent angle. Thrust your hips forward with your weight on the balls of both feet. Gently arch your back. Repeat Steps 2 through 4.

RANDOM THRUST

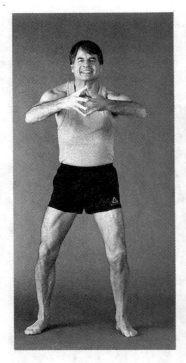 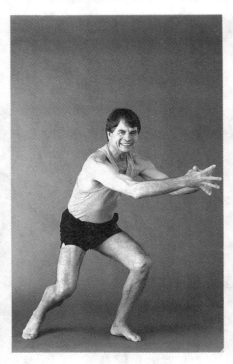 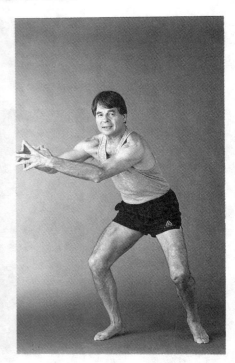

1

Stand with your heels 2' apart, feet angled out with your knees slightly bent. Push your fingers and thumbs together 8" from your chest. Hold your hands and elbows at shoulder level, fingers pointing forward. Inhale deeply before you begin.

2

Exhale completely as you push your hands with steady force out to your right until your elbows gently lock. Shift all of your weight to your right by centering your body over your right foot and bending your right knee. Keep your back straight and your head high.

3

Inhale deeply as you bring your hands back to near your chest without resistance and straighten your right knee. On the next exhale, push your hands with steady force out to your left until your elbows gently lock. Shift all of your weight to your left by centering your body over your left foot and bending your left knee. Keep your back straight and your head high.

RANDOM THRUST VARIATION

The Random Thrust is not limited to the instruction given here; it is done in both the pull and push hand positions. It is really a free-form exercise, where you can spontaneously take your pull or your push in any direction around your body.

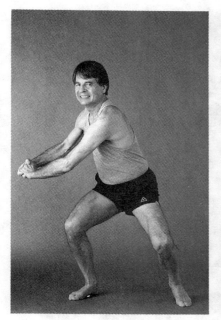
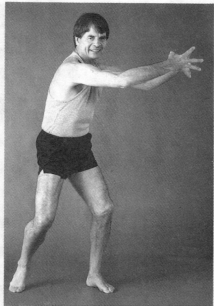
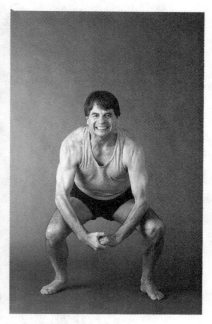

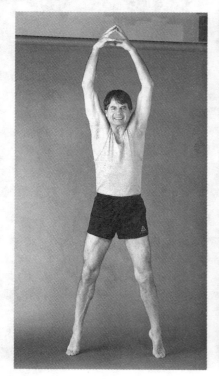
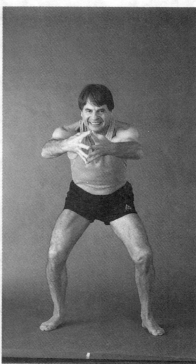

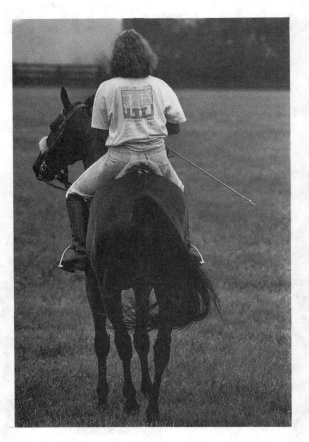
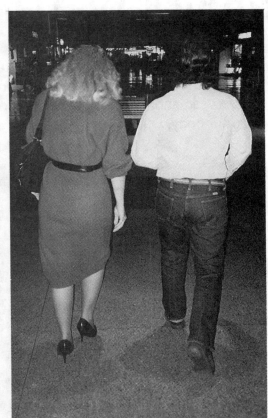
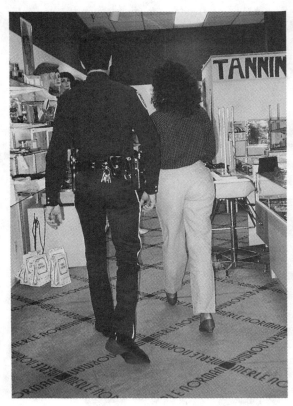
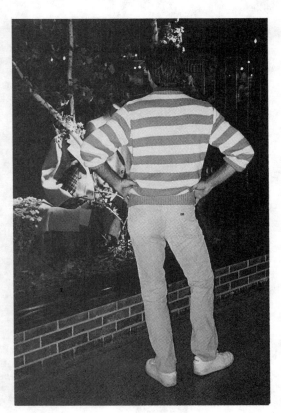

8

Synergetics Challenges

ADDED TONE—
ADDED STRENGTH—
ADDED COORDINATION—
ADDED FUN!

Adding Challenges to your Synergetics workout is like adding a special move to your favorite dance step or some extra spice to your favorite recipe. You are still performing the basic exercise, but you are incorporating additional motions that will challenge your mind and keep your body interested. Since they do not require any extra time, permanently blend as many Challenges into your regular Synergetics workouts as your body can coordinate.

Your behind is your first Challenge. It's unique! Nobody in the world has one exactly like it and since it is going to follow you around for the rest of your life, why not give it a little attention and care along with the rest of your body? You can reshape it and tighten it up with The Behinders.

By consciously tightening up one side of your behind as you shift your weight from one foot to the other, you add a major flex to your Synergetics motions. It's an exercise that you can do with every Synergetics workout and it's an exercise that you can do while you're talking on the phone, waiting for a bus, sitting in a car, watching TV, or anywhere that you are standing or sitting in one place for a minute or so. You'll learn how to flex your behind so that you will be proud to let it tag along behind you.

THE BEHINDERS

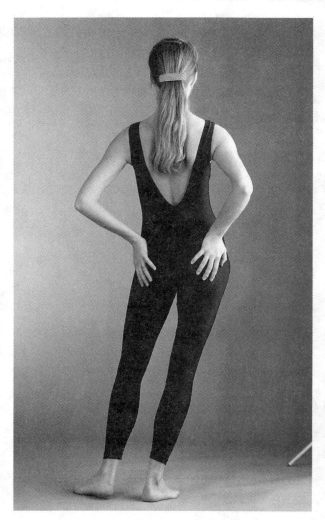 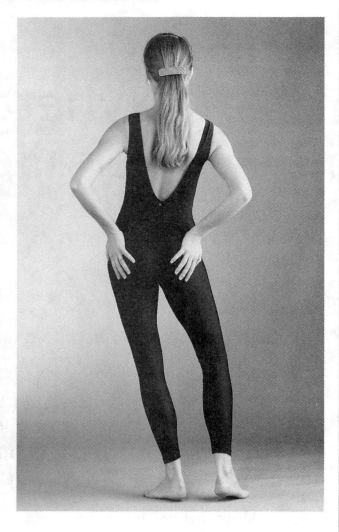

1

Stand with your heels 6" apart, feet angled out. Put your hands on your behind so you can feel your muscles tighten. Inhale deeply as you shift all of your weight to the ball of your right foot. Tighten the right side of your behind and the top of your thigh. Your right hand should be able to feel the flex. Keep your knees slightly bent.

2

Exhale completely as you shift all of your weight to the ball of your left foot. Tighten the left side of your behind and the top of your thigh. Your left hand should be able to feel the flex. Incorporate The Behinders from now on with every Weight Shift as you do Synergetics. Keep your knees slightly bent.

HEEL LIFT

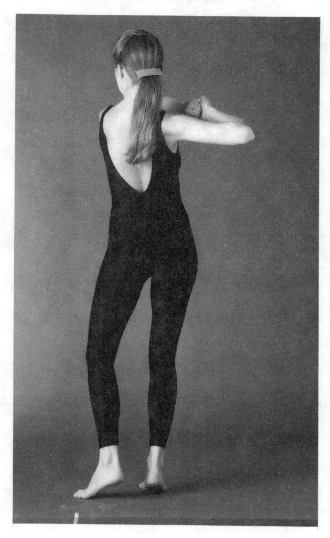

Here's a real Challenge for you. Hold your heels at least 2" off of the floor as you shift your weight, never letting them touch down. Keep your knees slightly bent with all of your weight on the balls of your feet. Keeping your heels 6" apart, feet angled out, staying on your toes, and never letting the heel of either foot touch the floor as you go through the motion will help you develop more balance and increase the strength and endurance of your calf and thigh muscles.

FINGER KISS

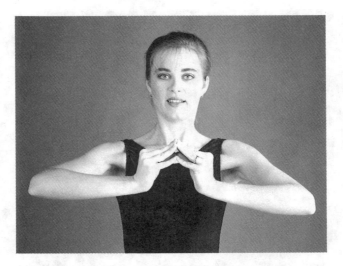

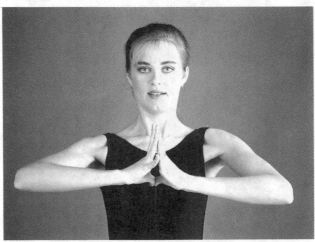

As you do a push (tips of fingers and thumbs pressed together) to the right, bring the tips of your fingers together until they are all touching. As you push back to the left, open up your hands (still pushing your fingers together with resistance) and spread your fingers wide, really stretching. This helps you develop stronger hands.

GRIP TWIST

With each motion, in every position, you can get an increased arm flex by twisting your hands through your pull or push. The Grip Twist is for strengthening your wrists, forearms, and biceps.

With the pull, slowly rotate your hands, twisting your wrists with resistance to their maximum as you pull in one direction and reversing the twisting motion as you slowly pull back in the opposite direction.

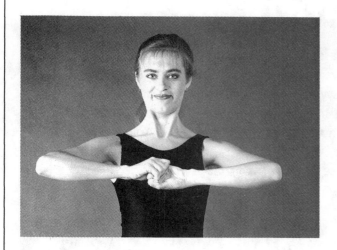 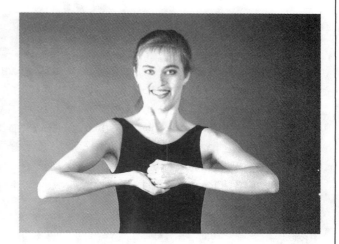

When pushing, slowly rotate your hands as far as you can at the wrist as you push through the motion. Reverse the rotating motion as you push back in the opposite direction.

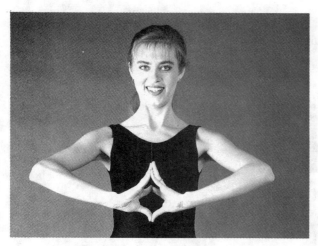 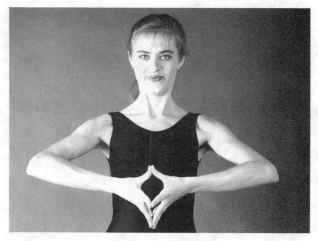

For an additional Challenge, reverse the direction of your twist, keeping the same breathing and motion pattern.

Take note of the additional action of your biceps muscles as you rotate your hands through the pull and push motions. Do this with every motion from now on.

BREATH SWITCH

Switch your breathing as you change from pulls to pushes or from one motion to another. Switch by doing two exhales in a row, which reverses the direction of your inhale and your exhale. This evens out your stomach muscle development by contracting your stomach muscles to the left *and* to the right and expanding them to the left *and* to the right.

GRIP SWITCH

You will be surprised at the new muscle combinations you can use by simply switching your grip. You probably always grip your fingers in the same way all the time without being aware of it. Try switching by reversing your grip—feels funny, doesn't it? One way seems natural, the other way doesn't. But you must exercise both ways to develop more hand dexterity and whole body coordination.

To switch your grip on a pull, reverse your grip so that your outside hand is the inside hand closest to your body.

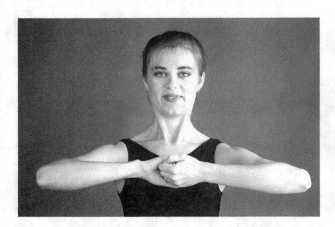 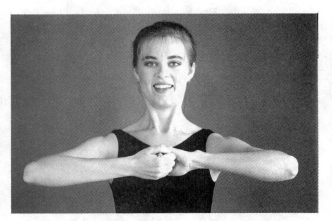
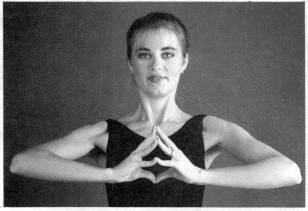 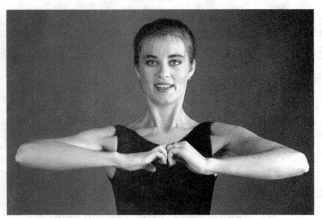

To switch your grip on a push, press your open fists together at the back of your first or second finger joints instead of pressing your fingertips together.

FOOT LIFT

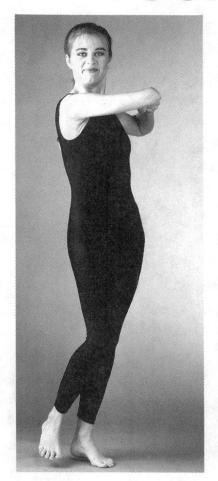 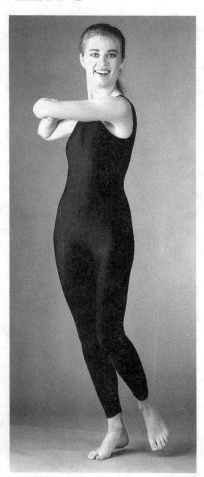

Each time you shift your weight from your right foot to your left foot, lift the foot without the weight on it a couple of inches off the floor. Now that you are becoming a pro at coordinating the rest of the Synergetics motions and Challenges, try the Foot Lift to improve your leg contour, agility, and balance.

BELLY SLAM

Inhale deeply as you pull or push to your right. Before you exhale and pull or push back to your left, contract your stomach muscles—pretightening your stomach before exhaling. Exhale completely with your stomach already tightened all the way back across the motion. This exercise can help develop extra power in your stomach muscles.

The **Double Belly Slam** is another super waist cincher. Instead of just exhaling once after you inhale, exhale again (without taking in more air) as you move the opposite way.

TOE STEP

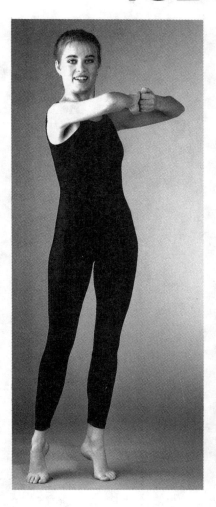 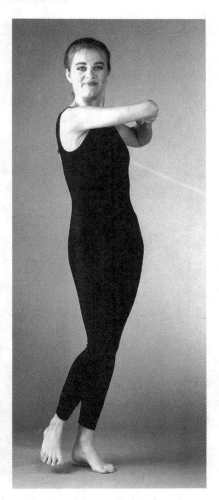

As you shift your weight to your right foot, raise your right heel high up so that your weight is on your toes. Hold for 1 second. Without lowering your right heel, shift your weight to the toes of your left foot and then lower your left foot until your heel almost touches the floor. Lift your right foot off of the floor. Keeping your weight on your left foot, raise your left heel high up so that your weight is on your toes again. Hold for 1 second. Without lowering your left heel, shift your weight to the toes of your right foot and then lower your right foot until your heel almost touches the floor. Lift your left foot off of the floor. This is an up and down motion that is great for developing balance and for foot and calf strength.

SUPER SLOW MOTION

This Challenge proves that "fast" isn't necessarily better. When you want to challenge your body for a real, honest-to-goodness power workout, go for Super Slow Motion with all of the resistance and control you can muster.

It takes a lot more conscious control of your muscles and a lot more endurance to do this kind of workout, even though it is done very, very slowly. Your body will have time to absorb a great deal more oxygen into its extremities with Super Slow Power Breathing.

Here's how to do it: With every exercise, exert extra pull or extra push and count 4 seconds (one thousand one, one thousand two, one thousand three, one thousand four) all the way to the right. Then count 4 seconds all the way back to the left pushing or pulling as hard as you can with a smooth, fluid motion.

BREEZING TEMPO

Breezing is a race horse training term meaning a pretty fast gallop around the training track. And that's exactly what you will be doing—Breezing with Synergetics.

There are four factors that you must watch carefully. Since you are doing *one flex per second* (twice as fast as the Basic Tempo and four times faster than Super Slow Motion) you may have a tendency to: (1) Swing, snap, or jerk your body back and forth, (2) Shallow breathe, (3) Forget to keep a steady resistance on your hands, or (4) Forget to stand tall. Consciously work to avoid all four of these factors. Why? Because (1) and (4) can injure your back and (2) and (3) can rob you of the benefits of your Breezing Tempo workout. This is a tempo that can raise your heartbeat up to fast jogging levels. So it is imperative that you absorb more oxygen than your body needs through your Power Breathing to help keep the strain off your heart and to help keep your muscles from cramping.

Here's how to do it: With every exercise, exert extra pull or extra push and count 1 second (one thousand one) to the right and 1 second to the left. Do as many, in as many positions as possible, for as many minutes as you can take. Breezing Tempo is the ultimate for building your endurance and your cardiovascular health.

Fast Mix: Try doing 12 minutes of Synergetics at Breezing Tempo without repeating any motion more than three times (any Synergetics motion done with Grip Switch counts as a different motion). Great workout for fast motion and fast thinking!

THE ULTIMATE RAINBOW

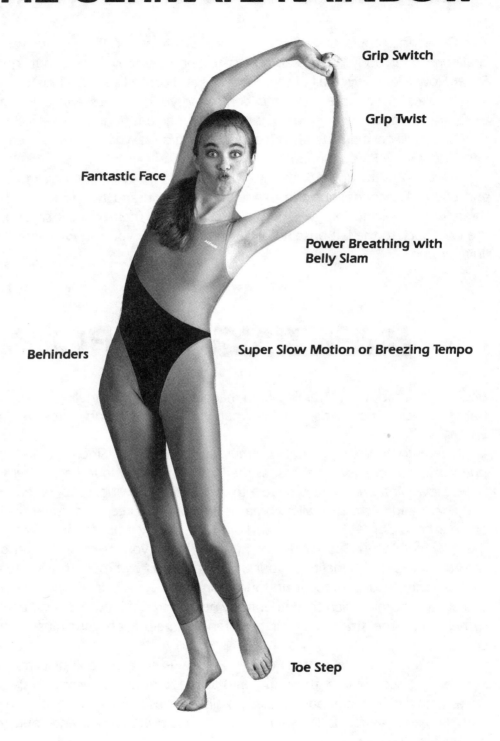

Grip Switch

Grip Twist

Fantastic Face

Power Breathing with Belly Slam

Behinders

Super Slow Motion or Breezing Tempo

Toe Step

The Ultimate Rainbow is either a Basic or an Extended Rainbow exercise which incorporates *many* of the Challenges, Power Breathing, and Fantastic Faces. This really challenges the circuits in your brain and all the muscles in your body in one motion.

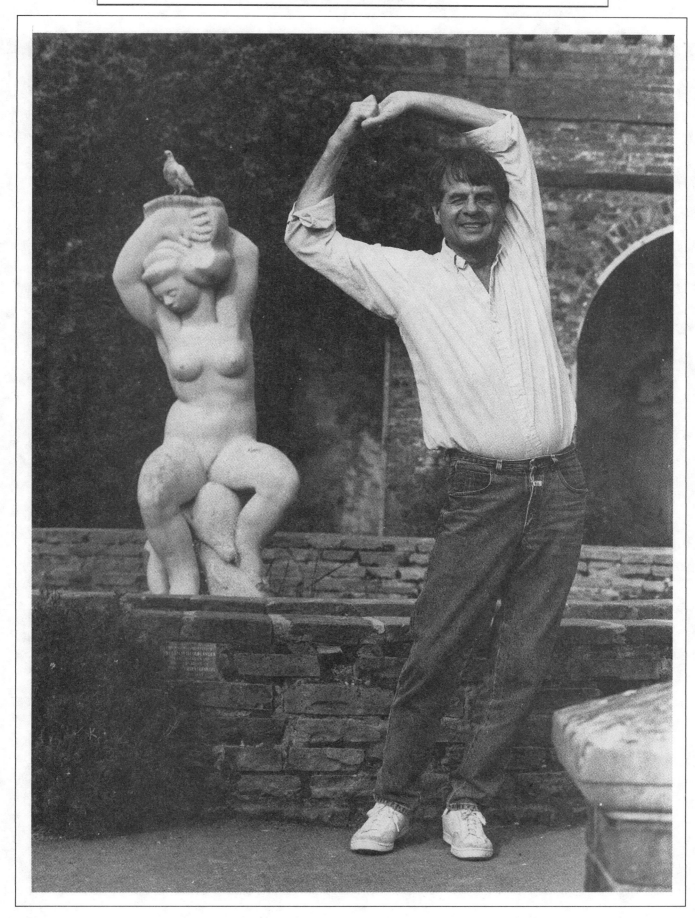

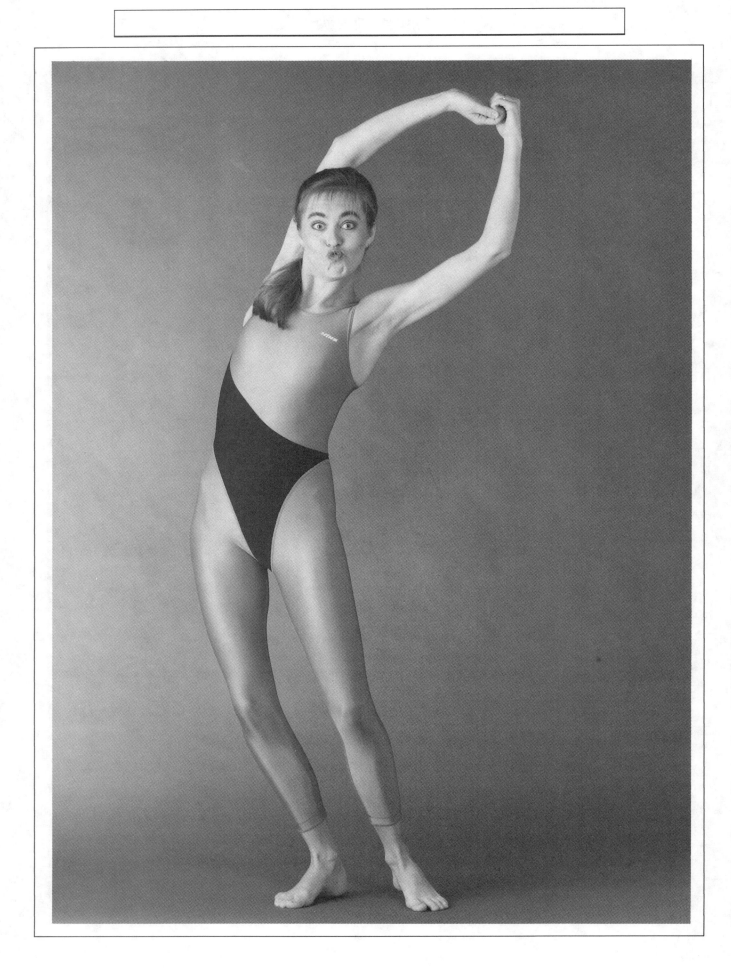

9

Synergetics for the Rest of Your Life

YOUR LIFE-LONG MAINTENANCE PLAN

Your body has now completed the full course of Synergetics training. You have the knowledge, but now you need the know-how which you get from *practice, practice, practice!* In several months you will look back and be amazed at just how little you were really using your body before you learned Synergetics. Make Synergetics a habit and you will become an expert on how to live a healthy, energetic life.

SUMMARY OF THE EXERCISES YOU HAVE LEARNED:

BASIC RAINBOW SERIES:	EXTENDED RAINBOW SERIES:
Chest-High Pull	Extended Chest-High Pull
Chest-High Push	Extended Chest-High Push
Low Pull	Extended Low Pull
Low Push	Extended Low Push
Overhead Pull	Extended Overhead Pull
Overhead Push	Extended Overhead Push
Behind-the-Back Pull	Extended Behind-the-Back Pull
Behind-the-Back Push	Extended Behind-the-Back Push

FANTASTIC FACES:

The Hunter
The Popeye
The Guppy
The Gorilla

POWER BREATHING

LEG SYNERGETICS:

Cat Stretch
Cat Stretch Variations
Stepping Out
Stepping Out Plus
Double Stepping Out
Stepping Out Heel Lift

HAND SYNERGETICS:

The Rooster with variations
The Hook with variations

POWER SYNERGETICS:

Pumping the Well
Stepping Out with Pumping the Well
Arm Wrestle
Around-the-World Pull
Around-the-World Push
Paddling Pull
Paddling Push
Paddling Low Pull
Paddling Low Push
Chopping Wood Pull
Chopping Wood Push
Random Thrust (Push and Pull variations)

CHALLENGES:

The Behinders
Heel Lift
Finger Kiss
Grip Twist
Breath Switch
Grip Switch
Foot Lift
Belly Slam
Toe Step
Super Slow Motion
Breezing Tempo
Ultimate Rainbow

Use this summary to develop your own daily program. Following are seven suggested advanced workouts. Each one takes approximately 12 minutes. You can use them every day or you can refer to them when you draw a blank in front of your mirror and can't think which exercises to do. You can stick with these, or make up your own personal workout program. The choice is yours. This varied approach to Synergetics will keep your body fit and keep your mind from getting bored!

WORKOUT ONE

Choose your own Fantastic Faces:

5 of each **Basic** Rainbow Pull and Push with at least 1 Challenge

5 of each **Extended** Rainbow Pull and Push with at least 1 Challenge

5 of each **Basic** Rainbow Pull and Push with Grip Switch

24 Cat Stretches Overhead (6 in each hand position)

20 Stepping Out right and left

WORKOUT TWO

Choose your own Fantastic Faces:

5 of each **Basic** Rainbow Pull and Push with at least 1 Challenge

10 of each **Extended** Rainbow Pull and Push with at least 1 Challenge

20 Stepping Out right and left

10 of one of the Power Synergetics of your choice

10 of another Power Synergetics of your choice

WORKOUT THREE

Choose your own Fantastic Faces:

24 Cat Stretches Out Front (6 in each hand position)

5 of each **Basic** Rainbow Pull and Push with at least 1 Challenge

5 of each **Extended** Rainbow Pull and Push with at least 1 Challenge

15 Stepping Out Plus Chest-High Pull right and left

15 Stepping Out Plus Low Push right and left

20 of one of the Hand Synergetics of your choice with variations

WORKOUT FOUR

Choose your own Fantastic Faces:

10 of each **Basic** Rainbow Pull and Push with Behinders

10 of each **Extended** Rainbow Pull and Push with Behinders

10 of one of the Power Synergetics of your choice

16 Cat Stretches Side (4 in each hand position)

WORKOUT FIVE

Choose your own Fantastic Faces:

20 of one of the Hand Synergetics with at least 1 Challenge
20 of one of the Power Synergetics with at least 1 Challenge
5 of each of the **Basic** Rainbow Pull and Push with Belly Slam
5 of each of the **Extended** Rainbow Pull and Push with Belly Slam
24 Cat Stretches Low (6 in each hand position)
20 Stepping Out with Pumping the Well to the right and left

WORKOUT SIX

Choose your own Fantastic Faces:

5 of each **Basic** Rainbow Series Pull and Push with Breath Switch
5 of each **Extended** Rainbow Pull and Push with Breath Switch
5 of each **Basic** Rainbow Pull and Push with Grip Switch
5 of each **Extended** Rainbow Pull and Push with Grip Switch
10 Stepping Out right and left

WORKOUT SEVEN

Choose your own Fantastic Faces:

20 Cat Stretches Overhead (5 in each hand position)

In Super Slow Motion:

5 of each **Basic** Rainbow Pull and Push with at least 1 Challenge
5 of each **Extended** Rainbow Pull and Push with at least 1 Challenge

In Breezing Tempo:

5 of each **Basic** Rainbow Pull and Push with at least 1 Challenge
5 of each **Extended** Rainbow Pull and Push with at least 1 Challenge
15 Stepping Out Plus Overhead right and left

THE MIRACLE OF SYNERGETICS

You have developed a unique skill! Anytime and anywhere you feel like it, you can join your hands, flex your body, breathe deeply, and fill yourself full of antistress, antihunger, and antiaging substances manufactured by your own body.

Let's review how you can use Synergetics anytime and anywhere you please so you can always keep a healthy balance in your life.

- The 1-Minute Stress Chaser—triggers body-relaxing endorphins and helps flush out stress related acids that cause a stiff neck and back. Do 20 repetitions (40 flexes) of your favorite Synergetics motion at the Basic Tempo, with Power Breathing and your favorite Fantastic Face.

- The 3-Minute Appetite Suppressant—triggers appetite-curbing brain substances (endorphins), increases your metabolic rate, and helps curb stress eating. Do 50 repetitions (100 flexes) mixing your favorite motions at the Basic Tempo with Fantastic Faces and Power Breathing.

- The 6-Minute Body Energizer—increases your circulation of oxygen-rich blood. Do 180 repetitions (360 flexes) mixing all of the Basic Rainbows at Breezing Tempo with Fantastic Faces and Power Breathing.

- The 9-Minute Brain Charger—delivers a good amount of oxygen to your brain and triggers mind-calming endorphins. Do 70 repetitions (140 flexes) of Extended Rainbows in Super Slow Motion with Fantastic Faces and Power Breathing.

- The 12-Minute Body Maintainer—increases your heart rate, stretches and tones your muscles, and stimulates the healthy function of your internal organs. Do a minimum of 180 repetitions (360 flexes) of the Synergetics of your choice at the tempo of your choice with Fantastic Faces and Power Breathing.

Design your own custom Synergetics programs. Fill in the blanks with your favorite exercise combinations. Develop several programs for your special needs and moods. Example: One workout for relaxation, one for a heavier workout. A wakeup program, a good-night program. Substitute one of your own workouts when you're feeling sluggish. Enjoy your special workout recipes just like you enjoy your favorite food recipes.

CUSTOM WORKOUT A

_____
_____
_____
_____
_____
_____
_____
_____
_____

CUSTOM WORKOUT B

_____
_____
_____
_____
_____
_____
_____
_____
_____

CUSTOM WORKOUT C

_____
_____
_____
_____
_____
_____
_____
_____

CUSTOM WORKOUT D

_____
_____
_____
_____
_____
_____
_____
_____

CUSTOM WORKOUT E

_____
_____
_____
_____
_____
_____
_____
_____
_____
_____

CUSTOM WORKOUT F

_____
_____
_____
_____
_____
_____
_____
_____
_____
_____

CUSTOM WORKOUT G

_____
_____
_____
_____
_____
_____
_____
_____
_____

CUSTOM WORKOUT H

_____
_____
_____
_____
_____
_____
_____
_____
_____

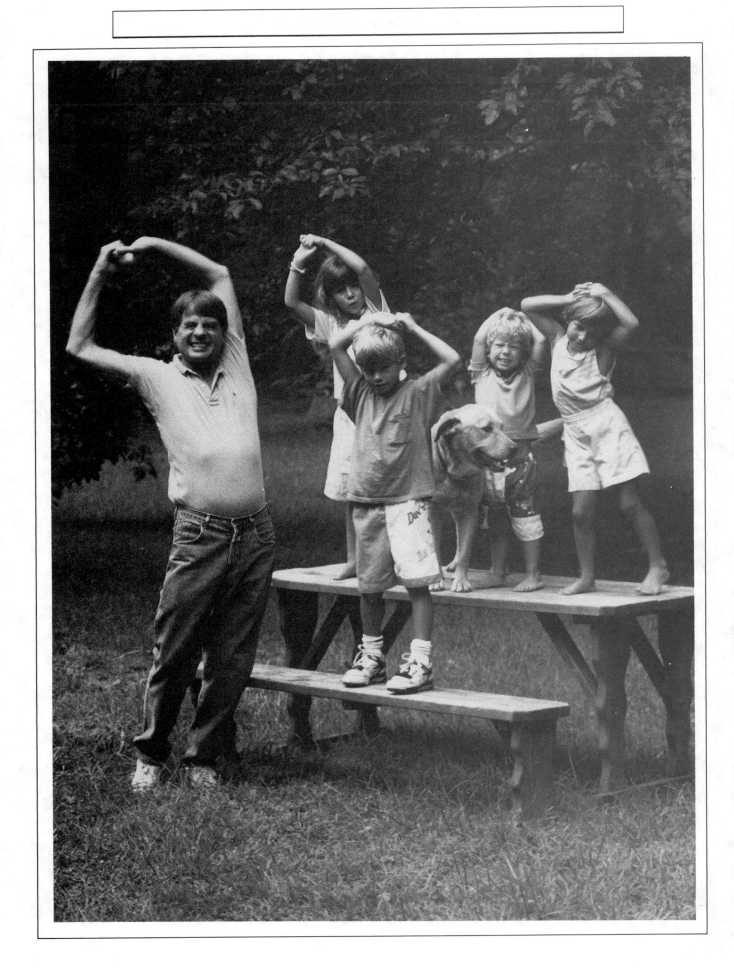

10

Any Age, Any Body

The purpose of this chapter is to give you a little insight into how Synergetics might fit into your lifestyle, whatever your age, and also to present some ways you might share this health system with your family, your friends, or anyone who may need some encouragement and help in taking care of themselves.

THE VERY YOUNG

It doesn't take a Harvard medical study to tell us when our children (and grandchildren) are not getting enough daily exercise. Just stand around your neighborhood convenience store and watch the children as they troop in after school for a candy bar or a cola. Too many appear to be overweight, sluggish, and weak. Their complexions don't glow, and their hair doesn't glisten.

Many schools have canceled their recreation programs for lack of funds and supervision. Children are literally locked in their classrooms. They are forced to sit, hour after hour, on hard chairs, without a break, and are expected to enjoy going to school, and to pay attention to what the teacher is teaching. Schools that provide recess and exercise programs for their young students have a much higher rate of learning, and a much lower rate of misconduct.

In a 1988 meeting in Boston of the American Association for the Advancement of Science, Dr. Rose Frisch of the Harvard School of Public Health reported that the benefits of moderate exercise for young girls "will last them the rest of their lives" by reducing the risk of cancer and diabetes. Dr. Frisch urged that girls, beginning at age ten to twelve, have at least two hours of team sports per week at school. Unfortunately, only a small percentage of children today get enough physical exercise or participate year-round in sports. Although this study was exclusively on women, it follows that exercise at a young age would also benefit men.

A southern Indiana schoolteacher is doing something about her children's present and future health: She gives her young students Synergetics breaks. The children do the exercises right beside their desks for five minutes or so in each of their classes. The children love the body movement, the Fantastic Faces, the energy boost, and the stress release. They are more attentive. Her class challenges the other classes to arm wrestling contests. Guess which class wins?

TEENS

Teenagers get even less exercise than their younger sisters and brothers. Driving around in cars replaces skateboards, roller skating, and bicycling. Munching popcorn and potato chips in front of television takes up hours of their day. Unless teenagers are very active, they may never fully develop their muscle structure and physical abilities. Many have no energy. They become listless, with a face full of acne and a body full of fat. They become depressed. Their bodies and their minds become easily stressed by minor challenges and changes. They become introspective and negative as their bodies go through upsetting hormonal changes. They often try to take the edge off of their stressful life with alcohol and drugs. Their schoolwork suffers, and they suffer. Many graduate to adulthood without the slightest idea of how to take care of their own health.

Much of this stress and frustration can be avoided if teenagers are encouraged to exercise, to feel proud of their bodies, and to develop the physical and mental stamina to compete in this very competitive society. Dr. Rose Frisch also reported in her medical study on the benefits of exercise for young women, that "women who played team sports in high school and college had a significantly reduced lifetime risk of breast cancer, colon cancer, cancers of the reproductive system and diabetes."

Parents can help by encouraging their children to exercise—by setting the example of exercising every day themselves, and encouraging their sons and daughters to join in.

TWENTY TO THIRTY

The time between the ages of twenty and thirty is often the most physically and emotionally demanding period of life. You're on your own for the first time. You begin looking for a mate. You begin your career. You get married. You have children. You are socially very active. You are trying to learn how to get along with your mate. You might have financial problems because there is so much to buy and so little money.

You don't get enough sleep. You aren't into routine eating. You do very little exercise unless you join a health club, but sometimes your schedule is too tight for that. You try to be everything you are advertised to be—sexy, smart, well dressed, educated, articulate, social, a good mother, a good father, a good provider—a superperson! Your life is a physical and emotional blur.

One way to make your body more relaxed and get rid of some of the blur is to train like an athlete! Up to about age twenty your body is a gift. After that you have to earn it! You have a choice of how you manage your life. You can go for the quick fixes of alcohol, drugs, and overeating to cover up the built-in stresses of your life. Or you can train yourself physically, mentally, and spiritually to use the built-in stresses of life as motivators for your personal growth.

THIRTY TO SIXTY

During the years between thirty and sixty, we experience a greater increase in responsibility. These are the years where we get so busy trying to make money and plan for the future that we forget to take care of ourselves. We have children who need to be put through college; we have to maintain a certain standard of living that takes all of our financial resources, and a considerable amount of physical and mental energy.

How many of your friends and family have you known who get so involved with their everyday life that they forget to relax, or even eat or sleep properly? By the time they realize (or are warned by their doctor) that they are in bad physical shape, they think that it's too late, or just don't bother to try to change. Many who do try to recapture their youth get discouraged by fad diets that don't work, or by strenuous exercise programs that they aren't physically capable of doing. With Synergetics you can adopt a reasonable schedule of physical exercise to help regain your youthful body and vital energy.

You can begin by making yourself your own best hobby. Look in the mirror and compliment yourself. Don't fret over how to cover up wrinkles, lumps, and sags with cosmetics and fuller cut clothes. Book time for yourself. That's right, for *yourself* that does not include anyone else. It's time for you to gather all of your being together, and love it just the way it is.

Exercise is no longer show business, it's serious business, and should be integrated into everyone's workday. Dr. Tenley Albright of the Advanced Medical Research Foundation of Boston urges that employers establish six- or seven-minute programs of daily exercise in the workplace to improve employees' health.

If you are presently working for a company that does not have an in-house exercise program, use your influence to get one started. Adults don't like to be tied to their desks and machines without a stress break any more than children like being tied to their school desks. Just like the children in a grade-school classroom who are allowed an exercise break, employees who exercise perform better and experience less illness and absenteeism. The health of our nation will largely depend on how much support exercise programs get in the workplace from the leaders of industry.

OVER SIXTY

When you retire, exercise is a real challenge. The lifestyle you have had for thirty, forty, or fifty years abruptly changes. The routines and priorities are altered overnight. Maybe you didn't take time out to develop hobbies and other personal interests. Maybe you focused on taking care of your family and your career. Your family has grown up now and scattered, your job is now done by younger people. With retirement you have more options than ever before. You are free! Free to study, to learn, to observe, to laugh, to relate, to savor, to share experiences, and to help others learn how to help themselves—but you must have the energy and good health to enjoy these good things.

You don't have to be biologically old just because you have lived a lot of years. Your body and brain have built-in survival mechanisms that will regenerate themselves—reaching back into the past to give you renewed strength and vitality if you just take a little time out each day to send them some Synergetics messages.

Everyone can adapt Synergetics to work with their special physical conditions. Even with large groups of people of advanced age there is rarely a person who can't do and enjoy Synergetics. One group of almost a hundred retired people worked with Synergetics for over an hour. The youngest was fifty-nine, and the eldest was ninety-nine with just a few in wheelchairs. Only one person sat down to rest before the session was over. She was ninety-three.

THE PHYSICALLY CHALLENGED

Some physical disabilities are minor inconveniences, but many require an entirely different lifestyle. Children and adults who are physically challenged may not be getting the exercise they need. With the help of a physician, anyone can create their own Synergetics fitness plan.

YOU COUNT

Whether you are very young or very old in years, it makes no difference. You have much to offer. The key to your life is your personal health and good feelings. When you feel good, the world is a wonderful place to be part of. When you feel good, you become attracted to people whom you can share with and help as you are helping yourself. Look for people who need help, who want help, whom you can help, and your everyday life will become a blessing—because the secret to happiness is feeling useful every day.

BRAINSTORMS AND ENERGY BURSTS

YOUR PERSONAL PROGRESS RECORD

DATE	WEIGHT	WAIST	HIPS	THIGHS	CHEST	STRENGTH (1–10)

COORDINATION (1–10)	ENERGY (1–10)	RELAXED (1–10)	SLEEP (1–10)

ELIMINATION (1–10)	EATING HABITS (1–10)	FACE (1–10)	OVERALL APPEARANCE (1–10)

OVERALL FEELINGS (1–10)   NOTE: Score 1 as low and 10 as high.

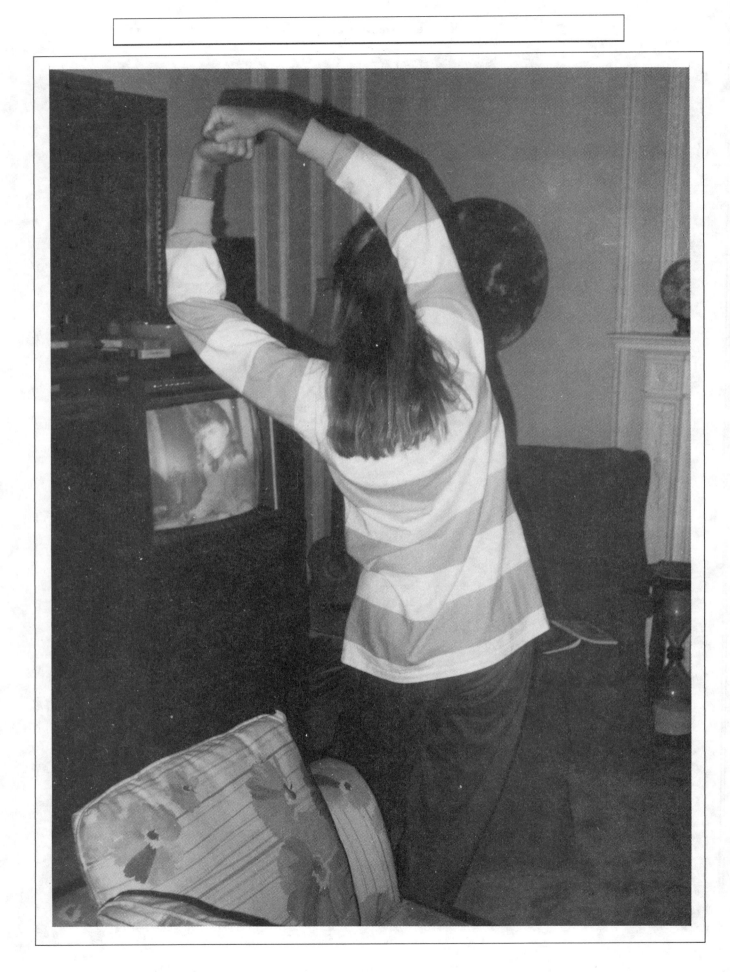

11

Avoiding the Major Agers

Your body is literally reborn every day. Billions of new cells are created by your body every twenty-four hours, and ninety-eight percent of your body is completely replaced by new cells every year. "New" cells, but not necessarily "healthy" cells. The health of your cells is determined by what you eat, by whether you exercise, and by your general attitude toward your life and yourself. Some scientists say that our bodies are equipped to live for 150 years in good health. That is, provided we can avoid the Major Agers: *Stress, Fat, Atrophy, Negative Thinking, Injury,* and *Hypoxia.*

Near Hilton Head, South Carolina, there is a small stone monument placed in memory of a tribe of Indians who lived along the coast back in the 1600s. The inscription tells how these Indians lived by fishing and gathering fruit and nuts, and how it wasn't uncommon for them to live in good health well past 100 years old. The inscription goes on to say that one member of their tribe had lived to the ripe old age of 165. It may not be possible for any of us to live to be 165 years old, but you can add a lot of healthy, satisfying years to your life by taking charge of your own lifestyle.

UNMASKING THE MAJOR AGERS

Think back to when you were a child, for a moment. You are in the playground, and you are holding on for dear life to your end of the seesaw. Your companion on the other end is a devilish little fellow, and when you least expect it, he jumps off of his end while you are tilted high in the air. Unless you were prepared to catch yourself, you came down with a crash, banging your tender bottom on the hard plank. If your prankish friend continued to "let you down" at his whim, you might not get on the seesaw with him again, or you may decide to find someone more trustworthy to seesaw with.

The Major Agers are very much like that mean little kid on the seesaw. If you seesaw with any of them long enough, you will come down with a crash. The trick is to know the names of these Major Agers and what they look like, so that you can avoid playing with them—ever!

The British philosopher, Herbert Spencer, once wrote, "The whole secret to prolonging one's life consists of doing nothing to shorten it." Don't let these "life-shortening" processes, the Major Agers, play in any part of your life. Let's see what the Major Agers look like, so you can recognize their deadly faces and avoid playing with them.

STRESS

Living Without Fear

Everybody has a unique set of stresses. For some, it's wild and woolly children careening around the house, or a problem getting along with a mate. For others it's the stress of career, or maybe financial reverses. With many, the problem is also what they eat or drink. Finally, there is the real and punishing feeling of not being accepted as we are—a feeling of not-okayness, or perhaps a fear of the unknown.

Stresses of all kinds are a part of your everyday life, and there is no way that you can run away from them unless you want to become a hermit and live in a cave. But there is a lot that you can do to see that the stresses that come at you don't hurt you. Good eating habits and plenty of sleep and exercise can build a shield of energy around your body. This shield of extra energy can give you the physical and mental power to transform stress into positive actions. When you are well rested and feeling good, you look at life a lot differently than when you are dead tired and physically shaky. Everybody has a different way of working with stress. Some whistle, some throw things, some laugh, some cry, some eat too much, some drink too much, some take tranquilizers, and some just go and hide in a corner. Why not replace these temporary fixes with the best stress reducer of all—*exercise!*

Living with a Light Heart

Let's go back a moment to being the happy kid in the playground again. Imagine that you have just stood up and brushed yourself off after banging your behind on the hard wood of the seesaw. You start to walk away, but something tells you that you should go back and try again. All of a sudden you get an idea! You will seesaw by yourself! You run back to the seesaw, climb to the center of it, and stand with one foot on one side of the center post and one foot on the other side of the center post. Very carefully, you test your ability to balance. Then, with a triumphant smile, you seesaw the plank back and forth by yourself, centered, balanced, and in total control. You're on top of the world, in complete control of the seesaw for the first time in your life! What a thrill! You yell over to your friends to look at you, and they want to try it too!

You have the power to feel and relish the joys that shower over you every day. A whiff of honeysuckle perfume as you walk by somebody's garden, the whistle of a bird, the laugh of a child, the sun warming your face, or the smile you receive when you tell someone you love them. Life is filled with beautiful things! You can savor happy moments like these every day if you choose.

Living with a Serious Mind

Begin taking charge of your own seesaw. Don't wait for something to force you to make a decision; instead make your own decisions, based on a more balanced, centered approach to your problems. Rather than planting yourself on one end of the seesaw, waiting for somebody or something to jump up and down on the other end, decide to stand in the center of your seesaw and move it back and forth to suit your needs. Like magic, the problems that looked so big before you took control, fade away.

A 1-Minute Stress Chaser

Since many stress symptoms settle in your neck, back, face, and shoulders, do 10 Low Pulls and 10 Low Pushes, 10 Overhead Pulls and 10 Overhead Pushes from the Basic Rainbow Series. Be sure to use Power Breathing with every motion, and get the stress out of your face with The Hunter or whichever Fantastic Face is your favorite. Dr. Gerald Amundson, a Chicago osteopathic physician, prescribes similar faces to his patients—stating that he believes face making is a natural part of our primitive stress release mechanism that has been suppressed by our social customs. You've probably noticed how children make funny faces to relieve their frustrations. You can do the same. This 1-Minute Stress Chaser can be done anywhere, when you can get a couple of minutes to yourself: sitting at your desk, standing in the kitchen, or riding in an empty elevator.

With Synergetics you will feel the stress leave as your blood begins to circulate more quickly through your body. Your shoulders, back, and neck will become relaxed as body-calming substances begin to flow. Your mind will clear. Your life will become fun again. Do your 1-Minute Stress Chaser several times a day, and feel the difference all day long.

Stress negatively affects every facet of your physical and mental being—aging every cell in your body and shortening your very existence. Be ever conscious of the subtle stresses that are splattering on you every waking moment, and keep on wiping them away without fear, with a light heart and a serious mind.

FAT

Fat's not bad. If you didn't have a certain amount of fat in your body, you wouldn't be healthy. But too much fat can shorten your health span and your life. In fact fat is the most visible and easy to recognize Major Ager of all. First, the facial features become indistinct as the fat cells puff out the cheeks and begin to form a double chin, then the arms become flabby. Finally, the thighs, stomach, and everything in between sags. Cellulite (fat cells that have broken through the natural netting of body tissue) begins to dimple the bodyscape. Larger clothes sizes appear in the closet. Breathing becomes more difficult. So does putting on shoes or getting in a car. These are the signals of a person who is seesawing with the heaviest Major Ager of all—*fat*.

Some people are more prone to gain weight than others because they are born with more fat cells, which the body feels obliged to fill up with fat. You can't safely get rid of fat cells. They are permanent receptacles which will attempt to store any fatty food that you send their way. However, you can keep them from getting fat with a regular schedule of exercise and reasonable eating habits. We inherit our body styles from our parents. We often inherit our parents' cooking and eating habits too, which can sometimes affect our health and weight even more than our genes can.

Eating Right

Irregular eating, like skipping breakfast or lunch, can actually cause weight gain. Your metabolism thinks there might be a famine coming, and slows down to conserve the food you have already eaten, so your body begins to burn calories at a much slower rate. Eat at least three evenly spaced meals each day to give yourself a good amount of energy, to promote regular elimination, and to keep your metabolic rate working at an efficient level. If you find you are constantly craving more food, it may be because your body is deficient in certain vitamins and minerals. Ask your doctor to recommend a good vitamin and mineral supplement.

Losing Weight

Gradual weight loss is more desirable than dropping weight too rapidly. Too much weight loss, too quickly, can shock your system, upset your metabolism, burn muscle fiber, and switch your body into a survival mode where it will fight back by forcing you to gorge yourself until it feels safe again. Gradual weight loss also gives you a chance to build up your muscles and retone your skin, while your body has time to adjust itself to reduced calorie intake. Your body's adjustment increases the odds that your new, more healthy eating habits will become permanent.

Timing Is Everything

"You can't lose weight with an exercise that doesn't make you sweat and burn a lot of calories!" This was the mythical mind-set of the eighties. What wasn't considered was that an exercise like Synergetics could conveniently be done at the two prime times of the day to burn fat and increase the rate at which the body burns calories— calories that are burned by the natural metabolic process rather than by the sweaty, "go for the burn" process. Two 12-minute Synergetics workouts done right before breakfast and right before bedtime permanently increase the rate at which your body burns calories twenty-four hours a day!

When you exercise right before breakfast, your metabolism (the body's system for breaking down food and distributing it to your cells) is awakened from a good night's sleep, and it immediately goes to work on the fat in your body.

In the study done by Professor Anthony Wilcox at Kansas State University it is indicated that in the morning your insulin count is normally at its lowest which allows your body to burn more fat. According to the same study on the effect of insulin levels (insulin is the body's blood sugar balancer), if you exercise in the middle of the day when your insulin level is high, you are mainly burning carbohydrates. This drains your energy and leaves the fat on your body jiggling for joy.

Your evening workout is done right before you go to bed, which again increases your body's metabolic rate, so that you burn additional calories all night long while you sleep.

Your Built-in Fat Stabilizers

Dr. Jeffrey Bland in his book, *Nutraerobics,* describes a natural and very healthy method of cutting your craving for food:

> Other substances that suppress appetite are neurotransmitters secreted by the brain called endorphins. These substances are also important for reducing pain. It is interesting that these substances are secreted after exercise, which may explain the appetite suppression characteristics of an appropriate exercise program. I am sure you've had an occasion when you've been famished and felt that you just had to eat, and then you got up to do something and you found that your hunger seemed to have gone away. Conversely, sometimes when we are the most sedentary and would seem to need to eat the least, we are the most hungry. The control of appetite by the secretion of appetite suppressive substances may be stimulated by proper exercise; a sedentary lifestyle will decrease their secretion and increase appetite.

Your most remarkable fat stabilizer is actually a fat itself. It's called brown fat, which is different from the yellow fat that it helps burn. Brown fat is a permanent, thin sheath of tissue that is concentrated around your neck and back. When you overeat, your brown fat actually heats up your body in order to burn excess calories. Ever felt exceptionally warm after an extra big meal? That was your brown fat activating its high concentration of minute mini-furnaces (mitochondria) that burn up those unneeded calories you just ate. Brown fat, like your body's muscles, can become almost inactive unless you do regular physical exercise.

As your exercise habit increases your body's muscle percentage, your body becomes a more efficient calorie-burning machine for reducing your body fat. Since muscle is more dense than fat, it contains more cells, which in turn, contain more of those same fat-burning mini-furnaces that will burn more of the calories you take in. The better your physical condition, the easier it is to stay in shape.

The expansion and contraction of your muscles plays an important part in breaking up fatty deposits too. The action of your muscles stretching and contracting across each other as you exercise softens hard fat that is locked in your body so that it can be flushed out by natural processes. The list of built-in balances that control the fat content of your body is too long to discuss here, but rest assured, if you are determined to create the body you want, follow this simple rule: Do more and eat less.

Don't be surprised if you lose inches before you lose pounds. Since a pound of muscle takes up a lot less space on your body than a pound of fat, you can drop several dress sizes or trouser sizes, develop curves and muscles, without losing much weight. This, of course, depends on your present condition and body style. Determine your best weight by how you look and feel. Don't go strictly by weight charts because those charts do not take your individual body type into consideration.

What you're looking for is a healthy amount of body fat and the ideal amount of muscle mass. The rule of thumb for women is 20 percent body fat and 80 percent muscle mass—for men 15 percent body fat and 85 percent muscle mass. This will vary from person to person and body style to body style, but it is a good standard by which to compare your own figures. The quick way to check your own body fat is to gently pinch the back of your arm just down from your shoulder. (This will give you a general idea.) If the amount of skin (and fat) measures more than a half an inch, you're on the wrong side of the ideal. If you pinch less than a half an inch, closer to a quarter of an inch, then you are approaching the ideal. More accurate measurements are done with calipers or weighing your body while it is suspended in water.

Eat What Nature Has Packaged for You

What you eat has a direct effect on how you feel and how you look. A healthy approach is: Eat food that is packaged by nature, and avoid those foods that are packaged by man. In other words: *If you can't peel it, crack it, or skin it, don't eat it!* Practically speaking this philosophy is a little too "rock hard," but you can keep it in mind as you stroll down the aisles of your supermarket and the piped-in music stirs you into a buying lust.

There are plenty of delicious foods that have no mysterious chemicals or added sugar. They might not be displayed as prominently as the high-profit junk food, so keep your eyes open. Eventually, you'll find that healthy foods taste better than the junk food; let your taste buds get used to Mother Nature's subtle sweetness and flavoring.

Life is meant to be fun and enjoyable, and nothing is more fun than celebrational eating. Why give up the pleasure? Even though we should all take our health seriously, we can still sample the "goodies" without becoming addicted to them. Changes in eating habits aren't going to happen overnight, but hopefully they won't take as long to change as they did to form. If you are old enough to read this sentence, then you have complete control over what goes into your mouth, and complete control over whether you exercise or not.

You don't have to make a big production out of doing Synergetics. You can do a quick series right before you eat, right after you have eaten (just as good as a brisk walk), and anytime you want to take the edge off of an urge to begin snacking. Instead of snacking during the commercial breaks, do some Synergetics. You will turn off your TV set in a lot better physical shape than when you turned it on.

Gaining Weight

If you want to gain weight, you can do that too with Synergetics. Do Synergetics twice a day and eat larger portions of nutritious food. The combination of daily exercise and increased food intake will activate your muscle fiber, giving it the ability to grow as it absorbs the additional nutrients.

ATROPHY

One of the quickest ways to age your body is to do nothing with it. Your body will only use as much of its muscle as you make it use; and if you don't use it, you will lose it.

Robert A. Anderson, M.D., in his book *Stress Power* notes:

I am frequently amazed at how quickly muscular tone disappears and tissue atrophies when a body part is immobilized. If a patient with a forearm fracture is placed in a long arm cast from the fingers to the middle of the upper arm for a period of six weeks, the muscle mass of the part of the arm included in the cast loses about one-third of its volume during that time. The arm, when removed from the cast, is weak and appears "puny" when compared to the opposite limb, due merely to the fact that the muscles involved have not been challenged or permitted to move for six weeks.

Many people feel that they are in fine shape—have had the same weight and measurements for years and don't feel it necessary to exercise. What they may not know is that their "high school" body has atrophied. The curves and muscle have been gradually replaced by semidormant muscle fiber marbled with body-aging yellow fat. Today's lifestyle of conveniences—riding elevators and escalators, sitting all day at a desk instead of chopping firewood, driving home with bags of packaged food instead of working in a garden—requires that we use only a fraction of our body's muscle. The rest of the muscle is just hanging there, getting a free ride on an underpowered, prematurely aging body.

To avoid atrophy, do Synergetics for 12 minutes at least twice a day. The more Synergetics messages you send your muscles during the day, the more quickly they will respond to exercise. Your body will not do any more than you demand. But if you demand more of your body than it is used to giving, it will create more active muscle to do the job you set for it. Well-conditioned muscle will give you more strength, more energy, quicker reflexes, and a new body form.

NEGATIVE THINKING

Mind Over Things That Matter

Along with positive physical messages you send your body every day, you must consciously practice sending positive mental messages too. It is the positive thoughts sent to your subconscious mind that govern the actions and health of every cell in your body. This mental exercise does not have to take any time out of your day, it can be done right before you close your eyes to sleep, and right as you wake up. You can also incorporate this same mental exercise into your morning and evening Synergetics workouts.

"Day by day, in every way, I'm getting better and better"—this is Emile Coué's general formula for preventing and curing disease. In the early 1920s, Emile Coué, a French psychologist, applied *Induced Autosuggestion* to the treatment of disease in his small clinic in Nancy, France. For years people from all over France filed through his clinic to learn how to apply Induced Autosuggestion to their own particular problems. People with asthma, tuberculosis, insomnia, alcoholism, nervous disorders of all kinds, miraculously responded to this simple little sentence. C. Harry Brooks discusses Coué's method in his book *The Practice Of Autosuggestion By The Method Of Emile Coué:*

> The Unconscious, in its character of surveyor over our mental and physical functions, knows far better than the conscious the precise failings and weaknesses which have the greatest need of attention. The general formula supplies it with a fund of healing, strengthening power, and leaves it to apply this at the points where the need is most urgent.

Brooks says that the use of the general "day by day" formula allows your unconscious to balance your personality without interference from some specific desires that might highlight a few characteristics to the detriment of others. He continues:

> Just as we leave the distribution of our bodily food to the choice of the Unconscious, so we may safely leave that of our mental food, our Induced Autosuggestion . . . the general formula leaves every mind free to unfold and develop in the manner most natural of itself. . . .

> Take a piece of string and tie in it twenty knots. By this means you can count with a minimum expenditure of attention, as a devout Catholic counts his

prayers on a rosary. The number twenty has no intrinsic virtue; it is merely adopted as a suitable round number.

On getting into bed close your eyes, relax your muscles and take up a comfortable posture. These are no more than ordinary preliminaries of slumber. Now repeat twenty times, counting by means of the knots, the general formula: "Day by day, in every way, I'm getting better and better". . . .

Say It With Faith! You can only rob Induced Autosuggestion of its power in one way—by believing that it is powerless. If you believe this it becomes ipso facto powerless for you. The greater your faith the more radical and the more rapid will be your results; though if you have only sufficient faith to repeat the formula twenty times night and morning the results will soon give you in your own person the proof you desire, and facts and faith will go on mutually augmenting each other.

Emile Coué's easy-to-understand, easy-to-use system of bringing the mind and the body together in self-directed harmony has been expressed over the ages in many languages and in many forms. Prayer, meditation, mantras, saying the rosary, chanting—all are closely related to this lovely, universal message from the conscious mind to the subconscious mind—"Day by day, in every way, I'm getting better and better."

Western science is now embracing what Emile Coué and Eastern cultures have known and practiced for thousands of years—that our minds control the health of every cell in our bodies. What we think is what we feel, and what we feel is what we are. Recently there has been an avalanche of new books written by Ph.D.'s, M.D.'s, and lay people, applying what they have discovered about this natural phenomenon called the power of the mind. There is now conclusive, scientific evidence that the energy of the mind can kill or cure the body, depending on its desires. An undisciplined mind is like an undisciplined child. He will deface the walls of his home with crayon, break the china, and maybe even strike a match and burn his house down. Our minds can get into this same mischief if we allow them to be influenced by destructive messages from ourselves or others.

Paul Pearsall, Ph.D. states in his book, *Super Immunity:*

Each thought and feeling is accompanied by a shower of brain chemicals that affects and is affected by billions of cells. This is our immune system, the constant surveillant of intrusion, of even the most minute malfunction of a cell within our bodies. The immune system identifies the invader, compares it to a constantly updated memory bank that knows friend or foe, and prepares an appropriate defense. It attacks the intruder, defeats it, cleans up after itself, and rids the body of wastes. While this is going on, the immune system learns, preparing itself for future challenges.

There is evidence that how we think is how we live. We have two choices: The first choice is living out of control with a fragmented, misdirected mind with high anxiety and ill health. The second choice is to teach our mind to take complete control of our own body's system so that we can live happily in excellent health for our maximum allotted time.

Advances in medical science have cured countless people of diseases that would have been fatal in Coué's time. But even with the great help of modern medicine, it is much more difficult to overcome disease without the cooperation of the positive mind of the patient.

Like wiping the squashed bugs off of your windshield every day so you can see clearly to safely drive your car, you can clean your mind and body of life-shortening trash by saying "Day by day, in every way, I'm getting better and better."

INJURY

Back in the seventies and right through most of the eighties, the Pied Pipers of strenuous exercise led millions of people into seriously injuring themselves. Torn ligaments, pulled tendons, crushed disks, sprained ankles, broken bones, damaged cartilage, pinched nerves—all damaging injuries that tortured the hopeful women and men who just wanted to stay healthy.

The Superman Complex

Excessive weight, force, or speed will sooner or later injure your body, and may do permanent damage. Most people consider their bodies indestructible—immortal— trying to prove that they can "take it" and show the world that they can lift more, pull more, and run faster than anyone else. What they don't know, until it is too late, is that the only person they beat was themselves.

When we try to keep up with some Olympic athlete type who teaches exercise for a living we can get ourselves into trouble. Many a poor, out-of-shape soul has been lured into an exercise studio, where Ms. or Mr. Universe shows off his or her skills by wearing them to a frazzle with 60 minutes of razzle-dazzle "cat-on-a-hot-skillet" exercise. After a few of these sessions, they limp home and make an appointment with a chiropractor or an orthopedic surgeon. A lot of this mad, mad, mad body-bashing exercise has ceased because of public backlash, but we still have to be wary of trying some exercise "just once" that looks a little too risky.

Numb, Numb, Numb!

Mother Nature took the necessary precaution of putting very sensitive nerves in most of your body so that it would "feel." Feel, so you can perform all kinds of hand work; feel, so you can sense where all parts of your body are in relation to other objects; and feel, so you won't unknowingly injure yourself. One place that does not have an early warning system of nerve endings is your cartilage, a spongelike, slippery substance that pads your joints against shock, allowing them to move smoothly against each other without pain. So you have no warning of pain or distress that you are destroying this absolutely vital cushion between your joints until it's too late. Unknowingly, a lot of joggers and strenuous aerobics enthusiasts are permanently mutilating their cartilage—the only padding that stands between them and severe, crippling arthritis in later years.

Cartilage, as we mentioned before, is the vital cushion that allows your joints to work smoothly, without pain. In its young, healthy state it has no nerve endings, but when it gets damaged by excess weight or impacts, it develops hairline cracks which then fill with scar tissue which has sensitive nerve endings—*causing you pain.* What this means is that when you feel pain in your joints, it's *too late,* the cartilage is already *irreparably damaged!*

So, right before you exercise, ask yourself whether or not the exercise you are about to do is going to exert excessive weight, force, or speed on your joints.

The authors of *The Rejuvenation Strategy,* René Cailliet, M.D. and Leonard Gross, explain:

> If 100 pounds of body weight is bearing down on your hips, knees, and ankles when you are standing, 400 pounds are bearing down when you walk, and 800 to 900 pounds when you jog. What [your body] doesn't need and cannot take is the pounding and grinding inflicted on it 900 times a mile whenever you jog. If you're an overweight jogger, the damage is that much worse.

Your joints may or may not be badly injured at this point in your life, but you should at least consider the long-range effect of any exercise you do from now on. It's never too late to change the exercise you're doing, no matter what your condition is. Synergetics can help stabilize previous exercise injuries, but you can never get back healthy cartilage and joints after they have been damaged. Work with what you've got. If walking is too hard on your joints, you can get as much or more physical benefit from Synergetics without the degenerating impact. Ask your physician to help you incorporate Synergetics into your injury recovery program.

When your joints go, you go. If you can't exercise, if you can't walk, and if you can't work because of unbearable pain, then your body will lose its will to survive.

HYPOXIA

According to Dr. Paavo Airola, "The medical evidence to the effect that ample regular exercise is imperative for optimum health is overwhelming. Exercise is absolutely essential to tone up your muscles, to improve digestion and metabolism, to maintain efficient nerve, lymph, and blood circulation, to prevent constipation, to assure the normal function of all organs and glands, and to supply enough oxygen to facilitate efficient cell and brain function. Keep in mind that the ultimate cause of premature aging is hypoxia, or lack of oxygen in your cells. The medical consensus is in complete agreement that our sedentary life contributes to many of our most dreaded diseases. . . ."

In prehistoric (and modern day) hunting and gathering societies, premature aging from hypoxia (lack of oxygen) was no problem. The clans or tribes all had plenty of daily exercise. The world's few remaining hunting tribes are virtually free of modern society's diseases such as diabetes, cancer, and heart disease because they eat healthy foods and are physically active. But what can we busy-all-day-working-at-our-jobs-and-taking-care-of-a-family do? The answer is simple—Power Breathing. That's right—Power Breathing. In addition to your two 12-minute morning and evening workouts, you can deliver a lot more oxygen to your oxygen-hungry cells every minute of the day by practicing Power Breathing. Over time, you can increase your intake of oxygen by a significant amount—an increase which will dramatically increase your energy, decrease your stress, and offset premature aging.

Start right now. Start inhaling deeply and exhaling completely with every breath from now on—for the rest of your potentially long and very healthy life. Consciously practice Power Breathing every chance you get—while you're doing your Synergetics workouts, driving your car, sitting at your desk, cooking your meals, watching TV, waiting at a bus stop, waiting for your flight or a friend, standing in the elevator, riding on an escalator—anywhere and everywhere you think about wanting to live younger and longer, until Power Breathing naturally becomes part of your life. Life truly is breath, and you can have much more of both by consciously breathing for your life from now on.

CHOOSE YOUR PLAYMATES CAREFULLY

Now that you have seen what the Major Agers look like—Stress, Fat, Atrophy, Negative Thinking, Injury, and Hypoxia—are any of them playing on your seesaw? The trick is for you to be superconscious of where they are, and how they disguise themselves, so that you can see them coming and take evasive action. It's going to take a lot of thought and energy on your part now, and conscious effort every day not to do anything to shorten the rest of your life.

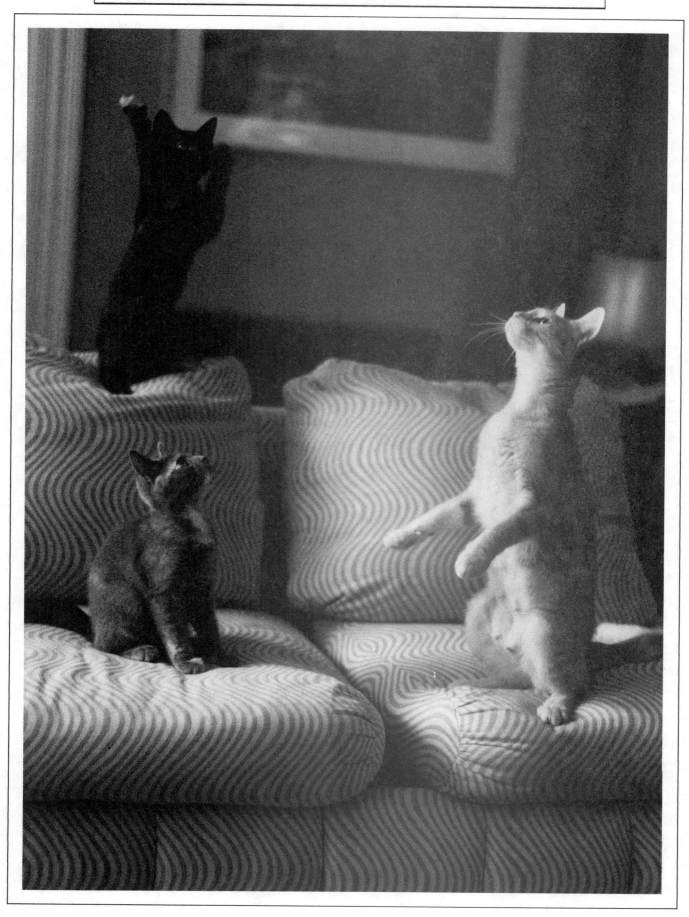

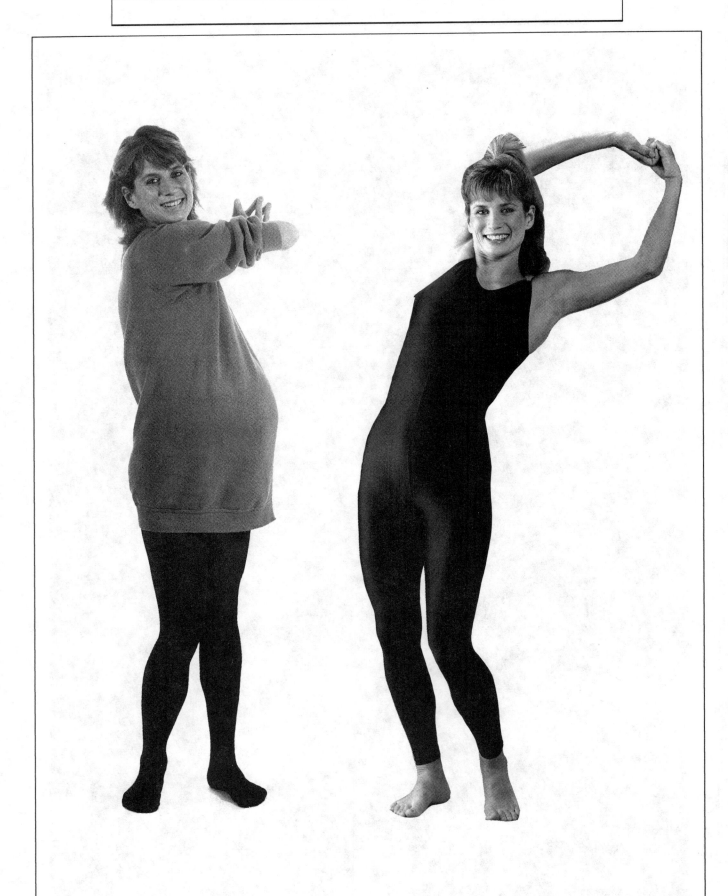

12

Fixing
Your Own Body

YOU ARE THE
MASTER MECHANIC

Mother Nature has never produced an imperfect body—only variations of her perfection. You have a perfect body now, and there has never been another on earth exactly like yours. Your body is unique in our carbon copy society, so you should be proud to own it just the way it is. But how good it feels and how good it looks is in your hands, so it is vital that you give it the daily loving care it needs.

Mother Nature didn't include a maintenance manual for your unique body when you were born, so you are going to have to write one for yourself. You can read all of the books ever printed on diet, exercise, how to think, how to look, how to get through your life, but none of the authors of those books, including the authors of this book, can know you like you do. So how can any one person or any one book give you all of the answers? They can't. You can, however, get a lot of insight, awareness, and encouragement from reading self-help books that interest you, and from consulting with the experts in the areas that you want to know more about. With knowledge and personal experience, you can decide for yourself what is good for you and what isn't—making your own conscious choices, and making yourself your favorite hobby.

When we exercise and eat well every day, and have positive thoughts every day, our bodies and our spirits do not have to age the way we were taught they should.

Our bodies can stay strong, quick, and beautiful, regardless of our age. We have the power within our own bodies to care for ourselves in perfect health, just as all living beings on earth care for themselves. You have a perfect body now, but you can improve on your own perfection by working every day with the most important person in the world—you.

There is no single thing that you can do to keep yourself healthy. Your body needs more than just good nutrition. Your body needs more than just the right amount of rest. Your body needs more than just a lot of exercise. Your body needs more than just positive thoughts. It needs all of these things—every day—in the right doses. Just as important, you need to teach your body how to avoid poisons hidden in commercially packaged processed foods.

This chapter can only give you quick peeks at certain health conditions, since most are extremely complex. We have selected the following subjects because they are common conditions and many are the focus of the fast-fix cures you see promoted on television. We have also targeted some of the most common food additives which negatively affect your body. Our hope is that after you learn a little about the causes and effects of certain health problems, you will use the information to either avoid problems or improve your present physical condition. Curing your body or avoiding an unhealthy condition requires personal action. It's really up to you.

BLOOD PRESSURE

There are many causes for hypertension (high blood pressure) such as obesity, stress, heredity, and diet, and there are many causes still to be discovered. However, we do know that regular physical exercise does help improve the health of the cardiovascular system, which in many cases will lower a person's blood pressure. By doing any kind of regular activity that increases your heart rate for a reasonable amount of time, you are going to receive some positive benefits. Working in the garden, a brisk walk, climbing several flights of stairs at once, frolicking with your children or grandchildren, running to catch a bus or a plane—all can get your heart beating at a rate which would be beneficial if you did any of them regularly.

Your heart is only about as big as your fist and weighs about a pound. It has to beat about 100,000 times a day to pump blood through 100,000 miles of blood vessels. If your heartbeat is sluggish, then this small but vital muscle doesn't get enough exercise. And if your blood vessels aren't healthy and clear of fatty obstructions like cholesterol, then your heart has to strain too hard to move blood, which will wear it out prematurely.

You must get your heart to beat at a faster speed several times a day—using its power to push your blood around your body more efficiently. Your blood vessels slightly expand and contract as your heart pumps blood. The brisk pumping action of your heart develops itself just as your arm develops itself by lifting weights regularly. The expansion and contraction of the vessels' walls keeps them resilient—able to relieve the pressure of your increased blood flow. The trick is to find an exercise that is sane enough and convenient enough that you will be willing to do it a couple of times a day to get your heart rate up to a level that will keep your cardiovascular system in good condition.

If you are an older person who hasn't exercised in years, you can do Synergetics at a slower rate—gradually building up your tempo and resistance as your strength and condition improves. If you are young and in good physical shape, then you can increase the speed of your motions, increase the resistance of your hands, increase the depth of your breathing, and increase the number of minutes you exercise to challenge your body. You can bring your heart rate up to the level of a fast jog without any of the impact to your joints. Power Breathing with every flex actually delivers more oxygen to your body than it needs for the action. This means that you don't get "out of breath" or endanger your heart by accidentally starving it of oxygen.

In 1986 The New England Journal of Medicine reported a study of seventeen thousand Harvard graduates directed by Dr. Ralph S. Paffenbarger Jr., a Stanford University researcher, which concluded that "you're healthy because you're active." The study showed that physical activity could counter some of the death-promoting effects of cigarette smoking, high blood pressure, or a hereditary tendency toward early death.

Walking is a wonderful heart stimulator and stress reliever, but because of time and weather limitations, walking sometimes becomes an off again, on again exercise. If you enjoy walking, and have a safe path to follow, walk a couple of brisk miles every chance you get. Be sure to wear sturdy, built-for-walking shoes and walk on soft ground whenever you can. Concrete sidewalks and asphalt streets are very hard on your joints when you walk. You can break up your walk with a short series of Synergetics if you choose, or actually do Synergetics *while you are walking*.

Two 12-minute Synergetics workouts a day can also serve your physical activity needs well, since Synergetics involves your entire body, including a conscious shifting of your weight from one foot to the other (giving you even more leg flexing motions than walking). Put particular emphasis on the Stepping Outs (or Stepping Outs Plus) and Cat Stretches, which can go a long way in conditioning your cardiovascular system. Since you sit so much—at the dining table, in the car, on the couch, at the desk—it makes it even harder for your heart to pump blood to your legs. Make a point of taking a break and doing the leg exercises during the TV commercial breaks, when you're on the phone, or just when you feel like your legs need a good flexing. The leg exercises will improve the circulation in your legs. Power Breathing can also raise your heart rate and stimulate your circulation. Try it for a few minutes and see how it works.

In addition to exercising every day, avoid foods high in fat, and excess salt and sugar. Avoiding alcohol, caffeine, and cigarettes is vital to your health, especially if you have high blood pressure.

CHOLESTEROL

In 1984 a study conducted by the National Heart, Lung, and Blood Institute showed that "the link between high blood cholesterol levels and heart disease is as incontrovertible as the link between smoking and lung cancer. The lower your blood cholesterol level, the better off you are; that much is sure."

There are two positive actions you can take immediately to protect yourself from too much cholesterol: The first is to modify your diet. Here's what the experts say in the June 1987 University of California, Berkeley "Wellness Letter":

> Whether or not you decide to have your blood lipids tested, there is a cost-free, trouble-free step to take right now, requiring no medical clearance and no lab tests, and that is going on a heart-healthy diet. The basic idea is to keep your cholesterol intake to no more than about 300 milligrams daily—the equivalent of about one egg yolk—and to avoid saturated fats as carefully as you avoid cholesterol. Fats should contribute no more than 30% of your total calorie intake, with saturated fats providing no more than 10% of that total. . . . Dr. Scott Grundy, a noted researcher in the area, suggests this as a way to postpone the coronary artery disease that overtakes nearly everybody after age 65.

Why all the fuss about cholesterol? Because it's a waxy, white substance—classified as a fat—that is guaranteed to shorten your life if you have too much of it in your system for too long. A certain amount of cholesterol is necessary for the function of your body (most of it is manufactured by your own system), but if there is too much, it will build up in your blood vessels until your blood flow is partially blocked. This condition is known as arteriosclerosis, which often leads to heart attack and strokes.

What is fatty food? What food is high in cholesterol and what isn't? Cholesterol is found in animal products—meat, eggs, poultry, fish, and dairy products. There is no cholesterol in vegetables, grains, and fruits. The way to improve your cholesterol level is simple—eat more no-cholesterol foods, and fewer high-cholesterol foods.

The second positive action you can take is to exercise every day. According to the experts, exercise increases HDL cholesterol (the "good-guy" cholesterol), which helps get rid of LDL cholesterol (the "bad-guy" cholesterol).

There is so much new information coming out about cholesterol, its effects, and its controls that it would be good for you to keep up to date through health newsletters and books. Take care to watch what you eat and take care to exercise. And, if you haven't had a recent cholesterol test, ask your doctor about getting one now!

OSTEOPOROSIS

In the November 1988 *Mayo Clinic Health Letter,* an essay titled, "Osteoporosis: The Silent Threat" concluded that by age 45 an estimated half of American women will have some form of this disorder. The Mayo Clinic essay describes the condition, saying,

> Bone is a living, constantly changing part of the body. Both sexes achieve their maximum bone mass by age 35. With age, and especially after menopause,

women's bones gradually become thinner. A decrease in the calcium content of bones coincides with the loss of estrogen. Doctors term the resulting bone condition osteoporosis ("osteo" = bone; "porosis" = increased pores).

The interior of bone resembles a sponge. With osteoporosis, the loss of bone seems to enlarge the "sponge holes," thereby weakening the bones. Osteoporosis is a "silent problem." It develops over many years. Often there are no symptoms until a fracture occurs.

In his book, *Wellness Medicine,* Robert A. Anderson, M.D. reports:

Moderate physical activity prevents osteoporosis. As early as 1892, increases in the thickness and mass of bone were shown to result from more weight-bearing activity, a response enhancing the ability of the bone to resist mechanical stress. The bone responds best to weight-bearing, antigravity, and strong muscle-contracting activity. Swimming is less likely to be helpful than other activities.

Your bones are like the trunk of a sapling tree: both need flexing in order to develop and maintain the strength needed to support themselves. If you leave stakes on a young tree for too long, it will not have the opportunity to flex in the wind which would develop its trunk. When the stakes are finally removed, the tree is malformed, weak, and easily blown down. If your bones do not get enough flexing on a daily basis, they too will become weak, brittle, and breakable. Your everyday activity is normally not enough exercise for your bones.

With the muscle extension/muscle contraction exercises of Synergetics, you are putting a good amount of flex, weight, and resistance on your bones. You do Synergetics by standing in one spot, without jumping around, with your weight naturally distributed on both feet. Synergetics is much safer to do than many other exercises which put too much impact on your bones.

The Importance of Calcium

When your bones are healthy, they are alive, strong, and resilient—like the trunk of a young sapling. They are fed in the same manner as the rest of your body—from your blood, which circulates through blood channels that weave through your bones. Just as a sapling must draw nutrition from the soil to develop its trunk, you must draw nutrition from your body to feed your bones. If you don't take in the proper balance of foods, you cannot feed your bones, and if you do not exercise regularly, the blood flow is not sufficient to deliver the proper amount of nutrients to your bones.

Your bones need to absorb more calcium, and a great source of *absorbable calcium* is fresh fruit and fresh vegetables. Calcium from dairy products is often difficult for the body to break down, and does not absorb into the bones as well as *water soluble calcium derived from fresh fruit and vegetables.* To get the most out of your fruit and vegetables, you can use a juicer to extract juices which are rich in water soluble, organic calcium. Do not overdo the juice; use it as a supplement to eating raw fruits and vegetables.

The Importance of Modifying Your Habits

In November 1985 *The Wellness Forum* quoted Karen Lutes, of the University of Louisville Department of Obstetrics and Gynecology. Lutes screens women for osteoporosis with a bone density scanner. She reports:

> Women achieve peak bone density between the ages of 35 and 40. If at any time you have a low bone density, there is still time to increase the bone mass through diet, calcium supplements and exercise. . . . At the end of the day, and if your diet has been insufficient, take a calcium supplement. It is also very important that women at risk for osteoporosis avoid smoking, alcohol, salt and stress.

> The article recommends a bone density scan at age thirty-five and then every five years until menopause. Following menopause, a scan is recommended every year.

> Synergetics is not the absolute cure for osteoporosis, but it can be a good step at any age toward preventing and treating the effects of osteoporosis.

ARTHRITIS

There are many known causes of arthritis of the joints—poor diet, overuse of the body, underuse of the body, and stress. Every time you stand, or even take a step, you are exerting pressure on your joints. Given enough time and enough pressure, your joints lose resiliency and begin to dry out and crack. There is also evidence that too little physical activity over a long period of time can cause arthritic conditions. What you eat can affect your joints too. A good example is gout, a painful condition causing inflammation of the joints—often the big toe joints. Gout is a condition commonly caused by eating too much rich food over too long a time. In other words, it is the result of a poor diet high in fat, salt, and sugar. There are also theories that some forms of arthritis are caused by virus and the imbalance of the body's ability to produce anti-inflammatory hormones. Much has been written about the effects of stress on the autoimmune system, which directly affects your anti-inflammatory system.

The jury is out on all of the causes and possible cures of arthritis, and to make any flat statements as to its absolute causes or potential cures would serve no purpose here. There are dozens and dozens of painkillers on the market that help relieve the pain a little, but the side effects of some of these pain relievers are worse than the effects of the arthritic condition itself. In the January 19, 1987 issue of *Insight* magazine an article was published titled "Exercise as Answer for Arthritis." The article takes both sides of the issue. One side contends that surgery is the best treatment for damaged cartilage. But a practicing rheumatologist has another view. He takes the position that exercise can aid in the treatment of arthritics by promoting the healing of damaged cartilage:

> John H. Bland, a rheumatologist at the University of Vermont, tells the story of an 85-year-old patient who was crippled by osteoarthritis of the hips. Bland did what he always does with his patients. He gave him quick lessons in the biology of cartilage and then put him on a fitness program. Within three years, the man was walking comfortably, and his joints continued to improve until he died at age 92.

> Such a remission from a crippling case of osteoarthritis is rare. Bland himself owns that, as a conservative estimate, only one of 40 of his severely afflicted patients has made similar progress. But he also says measures that on rare occasion cured those with severe arthritis can more frequently help those with milder joint problems.

If you have a problem with arthritis, ask your doctor about exercising with Synergetics.

ELIMINATION

There is one physical misery that television commercials haven't been able to exaggerate. You guessed it—constipation. There is nothing more excruciating than not being able to go to the bathroom. Since it is one of our most private bodily functions we usually suffer quietly, trying to smile all day through our "out of sorts" feelings. Improper elimination—constipation and irregularity—can shorten your health span and your lifespan.

Waste should leave your body just as quickly and naturally as possible. If you have chronic constipation, toxins from decaying food leak back into your body, causing all types of degenerative conditions. Countries that have a high-fiber diet— fruits, vegetables, grains—have a very low incidence of colon cancer compared to the United States where we eat so many refined foods and high-sugar products. The difference is that a high-fiber diet helps get the waste out of their bodies fast.

In his book, *Wellness Medicine,* Robert A. Anderson, M.D. reports:

> Denis Burkitt, a physician who served in the Public Health Service in South Africa for three decades, has widely reported that cultures with high-fiber diets had extremely low levels of serum cholesterol and incidence of coronary heart disease, compared to other cultures with low-fiber intake which exhibited high cholesterol and frequent coronary artery heart disease. A very low incidence of cancer of the colon and the entire gastrointestinal tract was also noted in tribes with high fiber intake. This may be due to the decreased transit time of food residues in tribes with high fiber intake. In western cultures with a high incidence of colon cancer, the average transit time is twice that of primitive cultures where the nutrition is very high in fiber.

An Apple a Day Plus Synergetics

Ho-hum! You've heard about the apple-a-day-keeps-the-doctor-away all of your life, right? It makes sense. Any type of high-fiber food has a positive effect on the elimination system. An apple is a real neat package of high fiber (be sure to include the skin) and most people like the taste. Tonight, right before you go to bed, slowly eat an apple, peel and all, chew it finely, and see how you do in the morning. Mix in 12 minutes of Synergetics with the apple tonight, and 12 minutes of Synergetics with a glass of water and a glass of fruit juice in the morning. The apple furnishes you a superior mouthful of fiber, and the Synergetics will get your circulation going as the motions gently massage all of your internal organs (including your colon). The water and juice will lubricate your digestive system, and get everything moving in the right direction.

The daily action of Synergetics exercises with Power Breathing gives your colon a gentle, internal massage that will help stimulate the circulation and vitality of your elimination system. Synergetics will also strengthen the muscles of the large intestine and your abdominal muscles which will strengthen the muscle contractions needed for efficient elimination. Be sure to wean yourself from any kind of laxatives as soon as you can, so that you don't lose your ability to function naturally for good.

Drinking water (distilled, spring, or filtered) is a great help for your elimination system. Water flushes out your system and also ensures that your kidneys are cleansed, to help prevent another type of elimination problem—kidney stones.

LOW BLOOD SUGAR

Millions of people in the United States have hypoglycemia (low blood sugar). One of these people could be you, and if you are suffering from hypoglycemia, it is very difficult for you to function energetically, much less have the energy and desire to begin an exercise program.

For decades, hypoglycemia has confounded medical science because it can masquerade as so many other diseases and conditions. Fortunately, the cure for hypoglycemia does not normally involve any drugs or surgery—only a totally healthy eating and exercise habit. So if you have any of the symptoms listed below, you may be able to relieve them by changing the way you feed yourself and the way you take care of your body.

In the book, *Hypoglycemia: A Better Approach* by Paavo Airola, Ph.D., N.D., the question is asked: Are you a victim of hypoglycemia? He provides the following list of possible symptoms:

• Do you feel tired all the time?

• Do you have to have coffee, cola, or alcohol to get you through your day?

• Are you forgetful, indecisive, irritable?

- Do you suffer from insomnia, depression, headaches, trembling, drowsiness, crying spells, cold sweats, mental confusion, anxiety, dizziness, indigestion, allergies, obesity, craving for sweets, lack of sexual energy?

This list shows some of the effects of refined sugar on the human body and reflects the growing need for healthy diets for every man, woman, and child in this country. The idea that refined sugar is a principal cause of much ill health in this country is no longer scientific speculation. It is scientific fact!

Hypoglycemia is caused by a malfunction of the pancreas which manufactures all of your insulin and distributes it to your body as it is needed to balance your blood sugar. The dietary cause of this condition is due to primarily overworking the pancreas by eating refined sugar in processed foods (the average American eats about 150 pounds of refined sugar each year). Drinking coffee, colas, and alcohol and smoking cigarettes also drastically affect the pancreas and the blood sugar level. Hypoglycemia can be the forerunner of diabetes, and getting rid of the symptoms in time is in your own hands and personal habits.

Walking the Low Blood Sugar Tightrope

You should avoid all foods and drinks that contain any form of refined sugar, caffeine, or alcohol. You should learn that there are dozens of deceptive names for refined sugar. Learn to read the labels carefully on the food you buy. You *must* eat complete meals regularly throughout the day—fresh fruit and vegetables, potatoes, rice, lean meats. Don't overdo it on high-protein foods or dried fruit.

Frequent, moderate exercise will help your body normalize its blood sugar level. According to Dr. Paavo Airola, most hypoglycemic symptoms are caused by oxygen starvation to the brain that results from low blood sugar level. When you feel that you are "going down," drink a little diluted fruit juice with a light snack, and do a short session of Synergetics, wherever you happen to be. Synergetics (include Power Breathing) can immediately supercharge your body and brain with the oxygen needed to offset many of the low blood sugar symptoms, and give you added energy to enjoy your day.

If you think you may have a blood sugar problem, see your doctor.

THE UNSEEN HEAD BASHERS

What do you do when you have a skull-splitting headache? Practice the piano? Play tag with the children? Balance your checkbook? Go for a nice walk in the country? Work out with Synergetics? Of course not. You run to your medicine cabinet and gulp down a headache drug, and dare anyone to raise their voice above a whisper. So, it's important that you don't get headaches all the time, or you won't want to exercise or do anything else positive for yourself.

Ever wonder where these head bashers come from? Stress? Yes, possibly. . . . What you eat? More than likely. Number one on the list is food shot full of different types of refined sugar products (and their aliases) which trigger a flood of insulin that burns up the sugar you ate plus more, throwing your body into "sugar shock" (insulin rebound). Number two, and not so obvious, is monosodium glutamate, commonly known as MSG.

Some restaurateurs tortured us by lacing the cuisine with MSG which prompted the *Wall Street Journal* to report that people all over the country were dining on Chinese food and then becoming short of breath, getting dizzy spells and heart palpitations, shaking, fainting, riding ambulances to hospitals, and *having horrible headaches that would last for several days*. The *Journal* dubbed this mystery malady "the Chinese restaurant syndrome." Several years later the truth came out: Chinese dishes were loaded with MSG, a laboratory-produced chemical that dilates your capillaries so that your taste buds are more sensitive to food (making the food taste tangier on your tongue).

Today, many Chinese restaurants are now offering their food with or without MSG, and some are not using it at all, but American-style restaurants and some fast food chains are using MSG on fish, chicken, beef, potatoes, and vegetables and in soups and salad dressing. Ask about MSG before you order or you may drive home with a queasy stomach and a brain-blasting headache.

Finally, a large percentage of packaged, canned, and "heat and serve" food products have MSG added. Read every label before you put the food in your grocery cart.

The reason that we mention sugar, MSG, caffeine, and alcohol is because they are serious body bashers. If you don't have any energy, and you have regular headaches, it will be very difficult for you to get into a regular exercise program.

NECK AND BACK PAINS

Many neck and back pains are caused by poor posture, stress, or imbalanced use of the body. Even in your teens, you begin to develop more muscle strength on your dominant side—the side of your body with the hand you normally use for eating, writing, throwing a ball, etc. Regardless of your age, you have a certain degree of overdevelopment on one side of your body that is pulling your body out of line. As you get older, your body will be pulled further out of line by unbalanced physical activity. Over 50 percent of the population has some type of back problem by the time they are forty, and 75 percent have painful back problems by the time they are 60!

The next time you are walking down the street, or shopping, or standing in line for a movie, observe the way people carry their bodies. Take a look at how many people carry one shoulder higher than the other, or that one side of their body is obviously more developed than the other side. The overdevelopment is often the result of unbalanced physical activity, and the hunching of their shoulders is often caused by stress. Their entire bone structure is misaligned, causing joints and bones to wear unevenly, eventually pinching muscles, nerves, and disks.

While you are "people watching," look to see whether they are standing tall or whether their bodies are hunched over. Poor posture has been recognized in Eastern

A message from Taylor:

Much of my inspiration and motivation to do more with my life has come from the encouragement of others—especially from testimonies of people who have overcome their challenges by taking action.

So I felt that you might benefit from reading a couple of e-mails that Joanna and I received—one recently and one last year that cover a lot of the physical problems that many of us have to deal with over our lifetimes.

I might add that we have received countless letters and e-mails over the past twenty-five years from all over the world. Without exception the messages to us have said in effect, that 'I have changed my life for the better by making Synergetics part of my daily routine.'

From: BCPonz
Date: Thu, 15 Jan 2004 12:20:01 EST
To: joanna@pocketgym.com
Subject: Synergetics program

Dear Joanna,

I just wanted to let you know how happy I am with the program. I started on Dec. 12,2003 and am faithfully doing the exercises with the power breathing. I turned 60 on Aug. 2, 2003. I suffer from neuralgia that effects my muscles and joints, especially my lower back and hips. My left hip was so bad that I experienced like a sciatic effect that went down my leg to my left knee, causing me to limp with pain. Medical tests show that I do not have arthritis, or rheumatism, or osteoporosis. I took myself off of hormone replacement two years ago after suffering bad side effects. These are now gone but I was very depressed.

About two weeks ago, all pain disappeared! I sleep well at night and have more energy during 0the day. Furthermore, I am not so depressed. At Christmas time I usually gain 4 or 5 pounds, but I maintained my weight this year. However, I did drop 4 pounds since Dec.12th and have lost a lot of bloat. My clothes are loose on me. I started the exercises to get rid of the pain but am happy to also bring myself to 115 pounds and maintain it.

Thank -you for making this program available to me.
Sincerely,

Beverly P

From: "k wolf"
Date: Sat, 25 Jun 2005 09:44:42 -0700
To: synergetics@pocketgym.com
Subject: Synergetics letter

Dear Taylor and Joanna;

Just wanted to let you know how very thankful I am for your Synergetics program. I can't believe the life I have gotten back, it's incredible!

   I am a 52 year-old nurse, and have exercised all my life. I have been in a few car accidents and mishaps with horses, (having lived on a small ranch) over the years. I've had a broken pelvis, herniated discs, smashed kneecaps, torn rotator cuff, and on top of that I participated in the North American Natural Body Builder's Association's amateur weight lifting and body building competitions. All of this physical activity, strain, and various injuries has led to deep tissue scars and a lot of stiffness. From all the years of abuse my joints and muscles finally began to give out on me. It started with arthritis in the knees from previous injuries added to standing and walking on cement floors for years as a nurse. I changed jobs and became much less active and very out of shape. At that time I began an aggressive exercise and walking routine to slim down and tone up.   I woke up one morning and the front of my legs hurt so bad (shin splints) I couldn't run and could barely walk. I could no longer do heavy lifting from upper and lower back pain from old herniated discs. I was starting to get panicked about the possibility of not only losing my job but of losing my
mobility. I became dependent on a cane for a few month's and was considering surgery to release the anterior tibial compartments in both legs. Needless to say, I walked and stood as little as possible for about eight month's. The more I tried to keep in shape with exercise the worse I felt. I could not even do the yoga I had been doing since I was 16.

   I read about your experience with Synergetics and decided to give your program a trial. This has been one of the best things that has ever happened to me. I have only been doing the exercises for a few months, but the change is incredible. I have my vitality back, and I feel and look five years younger. It's like the last five years were just erased. My legs filled out and have a shape again. My waist and bottom have slimmed down and I can now get into my "skinny jeans". I have strength and shape back in my arms, hands and back. I think I was beginning to lose the ability to break into a smile. The Fantastic Faces have changed that. My hair even feels better!

   I probably won't grow new knees, but I have learned to pace myself and relax into life. I never dreamed I could fill this good again, I thought that was behind me. Thank you so much for sharing this program with us.

Kristi W

health sciences as one of the greatest contributing factors to aging. Test this theory out for yourself. Purposely stand as erect and tall as you can and take a deep breath. Now, purposely slump your shoulders, allowing your chest to collapse down toward your stomach. Now try to take a deep breath. Can't get as much air, can you? The less air (oxygen) you get, the quicker you age, the more you slump over, and the more unnatural pressure you put on your neck and backbone. Your nervous system is pinched and every organ in your body has difficulty functioning. Not to mention that when you slump, you instantly look about ten years older than you really are.

Balancing Your Body

Atrophied muscle also contributes to poor posture. It's really difficult to stand up straight if you don't have the muscle strength to support your bone structure. Stand up for a moment, and look at yourself in a mirror. Now, relax your body and stand casually, like you do all day when you don't think anybody is looking. Get a hand mirror and take a look at the hump on your spine just below the back of your head. If you see it, that's a classic signal that your posture is not right, and that your body is prematurely aging. You may also be carrying your head forward which puts strain on your neck, and you may walk with a slight slouch (most people do). Your abdominal muscles may be weak, which leaves your lower back teetering back and forth, with very little muscle support.

These conditions can be reversed, provided you begin a regular exercise program that utilizes all of your muscles with equal exertion on both sides of your body. Synergetics works well because you work both sides of your body with equal force and frequency. The back and forth motions using pulling and pushing resistance with your hands can, in time, equalize the strength of the antagonistic muscles which hold your body in its proper alignment. Like the ropes that hold the mast of a ship straight and secure, your muscles must be strong and balanced to hold your spine, the mast of your body, straight and secure. If for any reason the muscles on one side of your body are weak, then your spine will bow toward the more dominant side of your body, and your out-of-line bone structure will begin to damage itself.

Stand tall with your body in a Perfect Posture as you do your twice-a-day set of the Rainbows. Your muscles will begin to develop themselves around your new-found posture so that you will have the proper support and muscle-strength balance to hold your bone structure in a healthier position. Within a reasonable time you will begin to notice that you can stand quite tall and upright with very little effort for longer periods of time. Practice the Perfect Posture suggestions every time you exercise.

Smoking is also suspected of contributing to chronic back pain called "smoker's back." In November, 1988 *The Edell Health Letter* reports an article in a 1988 *Nutritional Research Letter:*

> Statistics show that smokers have more back pain. . . . Now animal researchers in Sweden suggest that by constricting blood flow, smoking reduces the nutrients available to the disks in the spine. In a study on pigs, doctors measured nutrients in the blood, including oxygen and sugar. They found that after 30

minutes of exposure to cigarette smoke, there was a 50 percent drop in the amount of nutrients reaching the lower disks.

Stress is another cause of neck pain and lower back pain. In a time of stress we sometimes get into a habit of sitting rigidly, in one position, ready for the imagined fight or flight that never comes. The result of this do-nothing-but-sit-there-and-steam is an acid buildup in your muscles. This acid buildup (a by-product of metabolism) can't circulate out of your body fast enough, so it gives you stiff shoulders and a pain in the neck. When you catch yourself in an uptight position again, just take time out after the encounter and do a Synergetics 1-Minute Stress Chaser. Just do Power Breathing and do the Gorilla Fantastic Face. This action stretches the muscles in your neck, relaxes your eyes, and supercharges your body with oxygen and works out the acid buildup that kinked your muscles.

TMJ

Temporomandibular joint disorder (TMJ) has become a serious and prevalent problem for millions of people. Every time they open their mouths to speak, yawn, laugh, or chew a bite a food, they get popping noises and shooting pains as their jaw joint jams against the back of their skull, or the jaw muscles pull the jaw joint out of line in order to close. Chronic pain and headaches make life miserable. According to René Cailliet, M.D. and Leonard Gross, authors of *The Rejuvenation Strategy,* until recently this condition was thought to be caused exclusively by malocclusion, bad teeth, or irregular jaw formation. Now it is known that it is also caused just as much by faulty, "forward head" posture.

Cailliet and Gross point out that "forward head" posture is primarily caused by our everyday activities—doing paperwork at a desk, typing, working on an assembly line, cooking and cleaning—anything that requires that you look down for long periods of time. If you allow this "forward head" condition to exist over too long a period of time, you could permanently damage one of the most important joints in your body—the one you talk and eat with.

When you do your Synergetics workouts with an exaggerated, erect posture, you develop additional muscle support to offset the natural tendency to slump and lead with your head. Dr. Ballard Morgan of Lexington, Kentucky says, "Posture plays a prime role in positioning the jaw in order to rid yourself of the painful TMJ Syndrome. I recommend Synergetics as a convenient and effective exercise for developing the proper posture."

PREGNANCY

"I'm eating for two," should also have a companion sentence that says, "I'm exercising for two." If there ever was a time to start exercising, it's when you are pregnant. Your baby depends on you for everything while you are carrying it, and almost everything for several years after you have it. Carrying a baby can be a period of extreme physical beauty and joy for you if you are feeling strong and energetic.

Pregnancy is a time when you should be developing greater lung capacity so you can supply your child with more oxygen, both for development and during birth. It's the time when you should stimulate your blood circulation so your blood will deliver as much nutrition and oxygen to your baby's body cells as possible. It's also a time when you must develop especially strong muscles so that you can carry the extra weight of your child without injuring your own body. And it's the time when you must develop exceptionally strong abdominal muscles so that you can help deliver your baby quickly, naturally, and safely.

For the nine months that you are pregnant, and for quite awhile afterward, you are more vulnerable to injury than normally. You have to adapt to carrying the weight of a very heavy watermelon around your middle, which pulls your spine forward, making you awkward, increasing the possibility of back pain, permanent spine injury, and accidents. After your child is born, you have to carry him or her around on your hip, which can throw your back out of line.

Your legs and feet will sometimes swell from poor circulation and water retention, which also promote hemorrhoids and varicose veins. You run the risk of phlebitis (inflammation of the veins), as well as many other dangerous conditions. Your stomach muscles are going to be stretched, which can leave you with a permanently protruding belly. That's the possible bad news, but the good news is that you won't have these problems if you train like an athlete for the next nine months with the help of your doctor, and then make your training habit a part of the rest of your life.

Many women who adopted a regular exercise program when they got pregnant, ended up with a more beautiful figure *after* they had their baby than they had *before* they got pregnant! Carrying your baby doesn't have to age you one bit as long as you are willing to make the effort to exercise for two.

And while you are exercising for two, make sure that you *eat and live for two.* Eat the healthiest food you can find. Your body is giving up a lot of its own nutrition to nourish your baby, so don't take chances—be sure that you take a medically recommended nutritional supplement to assure that you and your child stay in perfect health during your pregnancy. Also remember that *anything* that you drink, eat, take, or smoke, immediately affects your baby as well as yourself.

Ask your doctor to help you design a safe Synergetics workout. Before adopting any exercise or diet program during pregnancy, you should consult with your physician.

PREMENSTRUAL SYNDROME AND MENOPAUSE

Millions of women are bashed every month by PMS (Premenstrual Syndrome)—cramps, anxiety, weakness, depression, and just plain discomfort. Then, in their forties or fifties, when they should be getting relief through menopause, their depressions and anxieties sometimes get worse. There are all kinds of over-the-counter pills and prescription drugs, and shots to help relieve the symptoms, but none of them can cure the cause. They only cover it up.

According to health experts, nothing can completely do away with the discomforts of menstrual cycles and menopause, but a good diet, no smoking, no alcohol, no sugar, no caffeine, controlling stress, and regular exercise will minimize the effects. You really have nothing to lose, and a lot to gain, by working with habits to improve the way you feel during these phases of your life.

WATER

A statement from the Environmental Protection Agency's report, "Lead in Drinking Water" concludes:

> Nearly 20% of Americans consume levels of lead in drinking water from public water systems exceeding federal standards for safety.

A 1987 *University of California, Berkeley Wellness Letter* article called "Wrap-up: Drinking Water" had the same disturbing news:

> In a national survey begun in 1974, the Environmental Protection Agency found more than 700 different organic chemicals present in water supplies in different areas around the country, including 22 chemicals known to cause cancer in experimental animals. According to a more recent survey conducted by Congress's General Accounting Office, 43% of America's 28,000 community water systems reported violations of federal health standards in 1980. Most tap water, according to the EPA, is likely to contain more than the recommended level of at least one pollutant.

The purity of the water we drink is vital to our health. Our bodies are made up of over 70 percent water and it's very important to drink at least eight glasses a day. It is becoming more and more apparent that the water available through our urban water systems is not fit for human consumption, or by any other living being for that matter. Our bodies need as few foreign substances in them as possible, and our cities' tap water is filled with chemicals and heavy metals that are causing health problems. Distilled water can be as pure as the glacier-fed streams that supplied our prehistoric ancestors. Our bodies were evolved on pure water, and they should live on pure water. Distilled water and some spring waters are excellent. There are also several home water-purification systems available. Think pure water, drink pure water.

VITAMIN AND MINERAL SUPPLEMENTS

Two time Nobel Prize winner, Linus Pauling, in his book, *How to Live Longer and Feel Better,* wrote:

My most important recommendation is that you take vitamins every day in optimum amounts to supplement the vitamins that you receive in your food. Those optimum amounts are much larger than the minimum supplemental intake usually recommended by physicians and old-fashioned nutritionists. . . . By proper intakes of vitamins and other nutrients and by following a few other healthful practices from youth or middle age on, you can, I believe, extend your life and years of well-being by twenty-five or even thirty-five years.

None of us is getting the needed nutrition from the food that we are eating, because much of the food available today is lacking in the nutrients that it once contained. Foods are grown on depleted soil, fertilized with synthetic chemicals, and stored for long periods of time before they get to us. From the time food is harvested, it begins to lose its nutritional value, so when it reaches our refrigerator, we don't know what vitamins and minerals are left.

We are generally overfed and undernourished. We overeat because our bodies instinctively force us to keep on eating until the vitamin and mineral deficiencies are made up (which they rarely are). If the food we eat is primarily "junk," devoid of nutrition, then the body wants us to keep on gobbling everything in sight, even against our wills—making us fatter and fatter.

The first step to losing weight is to *guarantee the nutritional balance of your body*. Do not deprive your body of what good food you are feeding it by dieting. Supplement your meals with vitamins and minerals that you can buy at your local health store. Try a basic multivitamin. Read about supplements and ask nutritionists questions about proper daily amounts. *Consult with your physician.* Use your body as your guide by consciously thinking about and analyzing how it feels. It's possible to become very draggy and toxic from taking too much of the wrong supplements. This is one area where it would serve your purpose to become an expert on what does and doesn't work well for you. Remember, your unique body needs a different combination and quantity of nutrition than anyone else's, so read your body's internal messages, and give it what it asks for. Keep it simple, but supplement!

ZZZZZZZZZZ

It's free, you can do it almost anywhere, it's fun, it makes you feel good, you can experience more exciting adventures when you're doing it than if you went to the movies, and without it you can't live. Come on, just for three nights, go to sleep no later than 10:30 P.M. and get up no earlier than 6:00 A.M. After a few days of this schedule, look at yourself in the mirror. The bags under your eyes are beginning to disappear. Your disposition is getting brighter. You smile more. There's a spring in your step and a sparkle in your eyes. Try it. Just tape that late show, do a few relaxing Synergetics right before you lie down, and have a new experience.

In his book, *Wellness Medicine*, Robert A. Anderson, M.D. reports a study involving 1,064,004 men and women done by E. C. Hammond, M.D. and published in the *American Journal of Public Health:*

In charting survival relative to previously reported hours of sleep, men having seven hours of sleep had the lowest death rates. The death rates increased for those getting more than seven hours sleep, as well as less than seven. Those getting five hours of sleep per night had very high death rates, and those getting 10-plus hours had higher than average death rates. Thus, it would appear from this extremely large statistical sampling that the optimum amount of sleep, relative to longevity and survival, is about seven hours.

Take a short nap whenever you can sneak, squeeze, or schedule one in. A nap can take the dip out of your day, and reenergize your body. Don't feel guilty either. You would be in good company with Winston Churchill, Albert Einstein, John Kennedy, and many other famous high achievers who were great nap takers.

Do a set of Synergetics right before you get into bed, to relieve muscle and mental stress—making sleep and dreams a pure and positive pleasure. ZZZZZZZZZZZZZZZZZZzzzzzzzz.

SELF MASSAGE

The odds are that you have never consciously touched or rubbed all of your body. With the index finger of your right hand, press down on the top of the wrist joint of your left hand as you open and close it. Feel the movement of the ligaments? When's the last time you felt them?

Wringing the hands is an unconscious, spontaneous way of relieving stress and anxiety. Hugging oneself is an unconscious self-protective motion. Pinching the cheek, rubbing the face, biting the lip, tightly crossing the legs, folding the arms, picking, scratching, licking the lips, are simply ways we unconsciously try to relieve stress in our bodies. Why not touch your body on purpose to calm yourself? Why not get in the habit of touching yourself all over every day? Go ahead, try it. You and your body will love it!

The benefits of self massage are boundless. You can get rid of stress, stimulate circulation, and improve your body tone and your complexion. Massage your entire body with a moisturizing lotion after your shower or before bedtime. There are a lot of books on self massage, and even little plastic cards on hand and foot massage that you can carry with you. Self massage is probably the most underrated self-help method around. Maybe it's because it's so simple to do and doesn't cost a dime. Give yourself a king's ransom of relaxation any time you choose—try massage.

SEXERGETICS

How do you rate sex? The greatest? The pits? Yahoo? Yeeeuuck? It all depends on your personal experiences. Sex is a very personal thing, and it can be an ongoing beautiful experience or a frightful chore, depending on the attitudes and physical condition of the partners. When you're relaxed and your energy is up, and your stress is down (remember that wonderful vacation?), your mind and body turn to thoughts of love.

Studies have been made on how we pick our mates and one idea is that there is still an instinct buried deep in our primeval memory that we should pick the strongest, most functional hunting and gathering mate we can find so we have a better chance of surviving as a team. The law of natural selection? Have you ever been attracted to someone who just seemed to have more energy? More radiance? More feeling of strength? Why take chances—why not get our hunting and gathering–style bodies in shape and see what we can attract?

Train like an athlete! Why not? Doesn't sex require athletic abilities? Sure it does. The more athletic you are, the more energy you have, the more you are going to want to participate, and the more energy you're going to have to enjoy it. Try Synergetics! It will do more for your sex life than a ton of powdered rhinoceros horn, and a vat of tequila!

BORN TO FEEL GOOD!

How many days in a row do you really feel good? We mean *really* good! If you feel good all the time, then you are a very rare bird. The average person has all kinds of aches, pains, discomforts, fatigue, upsets, and worries. The amazing thing is that most of our physical and mental problems are under our own control. Do you have any of the conditions mentioned in this chapter? If you do, then you have the option of getting rid of your problems by following the simple laws of Mother Nature:

Eat nutritious food.

Keep physically active.

Get plenty of rest.

You were born to feel good. Why not live to feel good?

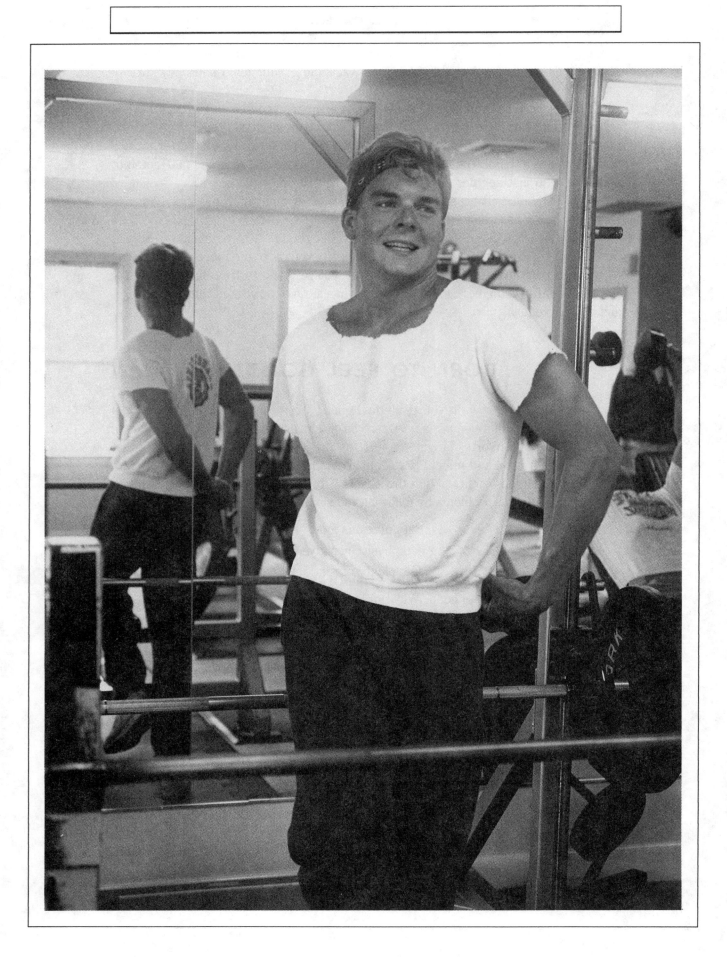

13

Building
Your Athletic
Body

What does the word *athlete* mean to you? A pro basketball player? A college football quarterback? A professional tennis player? How about: Anyone who does anything that requires a degree of physical skill? That could be a weekend golfer, an occasional tennis player, or a serious, highly trained athlete. This chapter is devoted to showing you how you can increase your athletic skills and cut down on injuries, whether you are a weekend golfer, an every-now-and-then tennis player, an exercise enthusiast, or a professional athlete. If you elect to play any sport or game, even once in a while, you owe it to your body to get it in condition so you can give the game or sport your best without getting hurt. And, even if you don't ever play a sport or a game, wouldn't it be nice to own an athletic body anyway?

I have often wondered whether I could have been a better athlete, a better football player, and avoided some of the injuries that I carry with me today, if I had trained differently. I think the only thing I would change would be to supplement every one of the sports and exercise programs with Synergetics. I wouldn't play any kind of game, or even use a piece of exercise equipment, without first warming up my body to its peak level with Synergetics. I wouldn't go to the shower without doing a complete cool-down with Synergetics first. In addition, I would discipline myself to do the regular morning and evening Synergetics workouts every day. If I had just given myself this extra training edge, I think I would have performed better as an athlete, and have fewer permanent injuries today.

Looking back, I realize that all of those exercises I did were really sports themselves, and that I should have trained for them just like I did for football. I was going to the local health club because I enjoyed being around other people, and I liked the challenge and relaxation I got from lifting weights, working out with Nautilus, and doing aerobics. What I didn't realize at the time was that my body wasn't ready for some of the exercises I did, and I should have trained, and warmed up, and cooled down, just as if I were playing any other sport. Since I wasn't training every day, my body never did get into top playing or workout condition. I was always sore for a couple of days after any physical activity, and hurt myself a lot because I wasn't in shape to make the moves.

Dance aerobics, weight lifting, Nautilus, jogging, running, golf, tennis, skiing, basketball, baseball, football, soccer, skating, horseback riding, bicycling—these are all sports requiring a regular training program if you want to perform well with a minimum of injuries. Whether you are a weekend athlete or a professional athlete, it's absolutely necessary that you continue to train and develop your physical abilities with something more than just practicing or playing your game. Your body is a resilient machine run by an immense computer that needs to be serviced with special types of activity every day to keep it in good working order.

If you play any kind of sport, you want an edge, an advantage over your opponent, the other team, or the game: graphite tennis racquets, high impact golf balls, superfood and energy drinks, special jumping shoes, secret plays, different grips—anything that will help you win at your sport.

But let's suppose that you already have the best equipment, and that you practice as much as your time will allow, and you're still not satisfied with your golf game, tennis game, basketball game, or whatever amateur, college, or professional sport you might be playing. Maybe you feel that your timing is off, or that you run out of gas in the final minutes of play. Or worse yet, that you are plagued by all types of injuries that take away from your ability to play your game. What you need is a way to train your body and sharpen your coordination every day, wherever you are, and anytime you feel like it.

BUILDING YOUR
OWN EXERCISE MACHINE

In a few weeks you can create your own unique exercise machine. It won't cost you a dime, and it has a lifetime guarantee. It allows you to exercise your body with infinite combinations of variable force, variable speed, in variable positions, and with variable ranges of motion. This machine challenges the limits of your strength, endurance, flexibility, and coordination. Its built-in computer instantly senses your body's changes in energy, and adjusts its force and speed to keep you from injuring yourself. It also senses any sore spots in your body, or potential points of injury, and instantly adjusts its force and tempo so that you don't accidentally aggravate the condition. This machine is so portable that you can take it with you wherever you go, and so compact that you can give yourself a full workout in the space of an airliner bathroom. You have always owned the parts to this machine. This machine is your own body! Use the Synergetics system to train your body to be your ultimate exercise machine.

THE SLINGSHOT EFFECT

Your strength and reflexes are determined by how fast you can simultaneously contract the greatest number of muscle fibers in your body on mental command. Pick up a rubber band, or if one isn't handy, pick up an imaginary rubber band. Now, stretch it as far as you can, and then let one end of it go. If it was a thin rubber band it went "snap," but if it was a thick rubber band stretched the same distance, it went "SNAP!" The strength of the snap was determined by how many resilient rubber fibers contracted simultaneously. The snap would have been even more powerful if the larger rubber band could have been stretched even further. This is the ideal rubber for making a slingshot—strong, with a lot of stretch and a lot of "SNAP!" Slingshot-type muscle is what you want to develop—muscle with a lot of stretch, and a lot of "SNAP!"

Another type of muscle is "garden hose" muscle. It becomes overdeveloped by doing too much weight lifting without stretching/resistance exercises to offset the shortening and bunching of the muscles. Grab hold of a piece of real or imaginary garden hose with both hands. Try to stretch it like a rubber band. Even though it is very strong and has a lot of fibers, the hose doesn't have the ability to stretch. So naturally, it doesn't have the ability to contract with a snap! Many athletes have this garden hose muscle—plenty of spot strength, but not enough quickness, or enough snap. Their garden hose muscle is just the opposite of slingshot muscle—stiff and slow.

Since the garden hose muscle is tight, even in its relaxed state, it tires quickly because the muscles actually get in the way of each other—they are muscle-bound. On the other hand, slingshot muscle is soft and resilient in its relaxed state, and when it is in action, every muscle is synergetically helping the action of every other muscle. Slingshot muscle is almost tireless and less injury prone because of its exceptional ability to contract and relax.

Slingshot muscle can be developed by using Synergetics because the motions flex every muscle to their safe limit with *maximum resistance* from your own physical power. This training teaches your muscles to work at a natural maximum load at their natural maximum extension. The longer the muscles become, the more snap they have and the more *power* they have. Since you are working your muscles to their maximum extension under *maximum load* you will also *increase the bulk and length* of your muscles.

Since many sports focus the entire motion of the body on hand action (swinging a bat, a club, a tennis racquet, shooting a basketball, tackling, dribbling . . .), it is vital that your training exercises focus your body's entire energy on the action of your hands. Every Synergetics motion is focused on hand action.

SUPPLEMENTING WEIGHT TRAINING WITH SYNERGETICS

Free weights, Universal Gyms, and Nautilus are excellent for building strength and bulk, but they are limited by the fact that the whole body is not used in real-life sports moves. Since all of these programs emphasize isolating certain muscle groups, and working on them while the rest of your body is semi-idle, your body doesn't get the opportunity to coordinate itself with repetitions of maximum resistance, and maximum range of motion while balancing on your feet. Synergetics can effectively supplement these weight programs and take up where weights leave off, by teaching your body to operate more efficiently as a whole, with your hands pushing or pulling against each other with maximum resistance, in various positions, to your maximum stretch, as you shift your weight from one foot to the other.

Synergetics will also offset the shortening of muscles caused by concentrated contraction workouts with free weights and Universal Gyms. Nautilus takes care of some of this bunchy, knotty muscle problem with "negative resistance motion" (allowing the muscles to elongate while resisting), but you are working in limited body positions with Nautilus compared to the positions you need to work with for your sports moves. By supplementing your weight programs with Synergetics, you can still build your bulk, and convert your spot strength to more functional strength with long, quick, slingshot muscles.

If you do a set of Rainbows every morning and every evening on your days off from weight training, plus a 12-minute warm-up and a 12-minute cool-down with the Ultimate Rainbow on either end of your weight workouts, you can add speed to your reflexes and more power to your body. At your option, add Synergetics for your hands and legs; this will increase their balance and endurance. For additional muscle separation and power, do repetitions of Power Synergetics until your muscles tell you that they have had enough. The increased repetitions of Power Synergetics will develop *holding power*—the ability to maintain the same resistance for a longer period of time and for more repetitions. And you don't have to skip a day to rest between Synergetics workouts, because they don't stress your muscles. You can do them as often as you like.

POWER PER POUND

Many sports do not require muscle bulk. Tennis, cycling, soccer, golf, swimming, many track and field sports, gymnastics, to name a few, require strength, endurance, and coordination but not necessarily a lot of physical weight. If you are competing in a sport that doesn't require bulk, then your goal is to be, pound for pound, the strongest, quickest person in the competition. The more physical strength and quickness ratio you have to your bodyweight, the better advantage you will have over your competition.

You can gain this edge in functional power-ratio to body weight by resisting the temptation to put on pounds of "show" muscle. "Show" muscle is "slow" muscle and you will get a lot more attention by winning than you will by body building. Instead of grunting around the free weights and weight machines, crank up your custom Synergetics power machine a couple of times a day and develop the extra percentage of power in the muscle you already have. You won't gain a lot of weight, but you'll gain a lot of first places.

THE QUASIMODO SYNDROME

Remember the hunchback of Notre Dame? This unfortunate soul was born with a deformity in his back that caused him to hunch over, and although the movie script writer didn't allow Quasimodo the lines to complain about the pain in his lower back, I'm sure he had plenty of it!

I have known a lot of semi-Quasimodos in my life—athletes who became deformed by years of overdeveloping one part of their body and neglecting the other parts. Body distortion happens in the arms and shoulders of tennis players, the legs of runners and dancers. It will happen in any sport or activity that overuses one or more parts of the body and underuses the rest. Many nonathletes suffer from imbalanced bodies because of overuse of their dominant side, but sports athletes seem to amplify this condition.

The racquet forearm of a tennis player is considerably larger than the arm that throws the ball into the air for a serve. Many players carry their dominant-side shoulder much higher than their less active shoulder. Even tennis players who use a lot of two-handed shots still seem to have an overdeveloped side. And when one side becomes more dominant, the muscles pull the backbone toward the strong side, pulling the body out of alignment, causing neck, back, and hip problems, and distortion of the body.

A distance runner once told me that her upper body gave out before her legs did. Most of her training was concentrated on her legs, with little attention paid to her torso. The result was that her overtrained legs were robbing her upper body of the necessary protein to maintain its muscle and endurance. This same condition is also pronounced in ballet dancers. Years of dancing overdevelops the legs and ignores the upper body, which is often not given enough exercise to keep up.

Sweden is trying to help runners develop the rest of their bodies by placing exercise stations at regular intervals on running courses. The runners can stop and work through an exercise routine—chinning, climbing, etc.—that helps develop other parts of their bodies.

You can chart a similar course for yourself and make Synergetics stops which will give you some of the benefits of the Swedish exercise stations. Walkers who want additional body training can also make periodic Synergetics stops, or do upper body Synergetics as they walk.

Training with Synergetics can compensate for overdevelopment from the overuse of one side, and gradually bring an athlete's body back into alignment. The equalized back and forth motions with strong resistance will allow the weak side to become almost equal to the dominant side in strength and dexterity. It is very important that you don't carry unnecessary battle scars and pain with you for the rest of your life just because you didn't train properly for your few early years of strenuous athletics. By taking the little extra time to do a Synergetics workout to balance and tune your body before you work out with your sport, you can add years to your playing career and years to your body's health.

YOUR BUILT-IN OSCILLATING BEAM

An oscillating beam is an easily tilted platform which requires that you balance yourself as you go through your sports motions. By performing a full range of exercises and sports motions, like swinging a tennis racquet or a bat, as you balance on the teetering board, you can increase your ability to balance, move, swing, and perform your sports moves.

You can effectively duplicate this oscillating beam exercise and train your body for your sports moves by working out daily with the Rainbow Series in combination with the Toe Step technique. This technique trains your body to work on the toes of one foot (like a ballet dancer), and maintain the power and eye-hand coordination needed to perform efficient sports moves. In addition, the Toe Step technique trains the muscles of your legs to better handle the variable impacts and motions of your sports moves.

BREATH SWITCH

Practice the Breath Switch with your Synergetics workout, so that you can make all of your sports moves just as efficiently whether you are inhaling or exhaling on the move. Since your reflexes can be faster than the time it takes you to inhale, it would help to learn how to make your sports moves just as efficiently whether you are inhaling or exhaling at the time. Practice exhaling on the backswing of your tennis stroke as well as inhaling. There will be times when you have to change direction, adjust your body, and make your move faster than you can switch your breathing pattern. Having to inhale first to make a certain move can sometimes lessen the effectiveness of a move, so practice making your moves and taking your shots with the Breath Switch to improve your performance.

GRIP SWITCH FOR TWO-HANDED DEXTERITY

Switch hitters, those who can hit a baseball right-handed or left-handed, passers who can throw the football with either hand, basketball players who can shoot, dribble, or pass just as effectively with either hand, can be more valuable than one-sided athletes. The Grip Switch trains an entirely different combination of muscles to work together—doing the same motions, but using your less dominant side as the lead hand. Always do half of your Synergetics with your less dominant grip. These motions will train your brain and body to cross over and make moves that you originally trained only your dominant hand to do.

REPETITIONS FOR
COORDINATION AND ENDURANCE

If you just do Synergetics for 12 minutes, twice a day, and do them slowly (one flex every 2 seconds), you are doing 720 flexes a day. Multiply that by seven and you've done 5040 a week times fifty-two is 262,080 a year! In ten years, that's well over 2 million Synergetics flexes. If you do your Synergetics at the Breezing Tempo, then you are doubling the number of flexes you do.

This many repetitions of almost any other exercise program would stress your body beyond repair, but Synergetics motions don't hurt you—they strengthen and keep your body flexible. Synergetics are *no-impact* exercises that exert your body in its most natural, upright stance, so there is no excessive wear on your joints.

For endurance training, increase the number of repetitions in each position of the Rainbow Series with two types of action: For strength, do the Rainbow Series and selected Power Synergetics in Super Slow Motion (one flex every 4 seconds)—with all the strength you have. For endurance, do the Rainbow Series and selected Power Synergetics in Breezing Tempo (one flex per second), and increase your nonstop series a minimum of 18 minutes at a time rather than 12 minutes. After a few months of this training, you will have fewer problems with arm weariness and slowed reflexes.

POWER BREATHING
FOR ENDURANCE

The Synergetics method of Power Breathing trains you to consciously force oxygen into your body so that your body gets a greater volume of oxygen to give you extra energy and endurance—and fewer injuries. You can do a series of Breezing Tempo motions for however many minutes you choose, with your maximum hand resistance, and not be out of breath at the end of your workout—*provided you use Power Breathing* with every motion. Your heart is smoothly racing along on oxygen-rich blood, getting a safe cardiovascular workout, instead of frantically beating to get oxygen from oxygen-starved blood. You can test the effectiveness of your Power Breathing by doing your workout, then stopping to carry on a normal conversation for 15 to 20 seconds before you have to pause for another breath.

THE POWER OF
SYNERGETICS IMAGING

It may be that you can improve your sports performance by adding Synergetics Imaging to your training program. Synergetics Imaging is a technique which combines training motions that resemble your sports moves with mental imaging. The training involves muscle-control exercises which are done in a very slow, consciously controlled, coordinated motion, as you imagine that you are actually playing your game.

This mental power is described in *The Practice of Autosuggestion by the Method of Emile Coué,* where the author, C. Harry Brooks, quotes Coué:

> Success is not gained by effort but by right thinking. The champion golfer or tennis-player is not a person of herculean frame and immense will-power. His whole life has been dominated by the thought of success in the game at which he excels.

Mental imaging to improve sports performance is nothing new. In his book, *Psycho-Cybernetics,* Maxwell Maltz, M.D., F.I.C.S. writes:

> Mental pictures offer us an opportunity to "practice" new traits and attitudes, which otherwise we could not do. This is possible because your nervous system cannot tell the difference between an actual experience and one that is vividly imagined.

Dr. Maltz cites a study reported in *Research Quarterly* demonstrating this point. It was done by selecting three random groups of people to shoot basketball free throws. Each group shot at the goal and their scores were tallied. The first group was told to come back in 20 days for another test, but not to practice at all. The second group was told to practice every day for 20 minutes actually shooting free throws for 20 days, and then to come back for a test. The third group was sent home with the instructions to not practice, but to sit in a chair every day for 20 minutes, imagining, with their eyes closed, that they were shooting at the basketball goal and making their shots, and then come back in 20 days for a test.

At the end of 20 days, the group that physically practiced for 20 minutes a day, increased their performance by 24 percent. The group that didn't do anything for 20 days didn't improve. But, the group that sat in a chair imagining that they were shooting free throws every day for 20 minutes, increased their shooting percentage by 23 percent! Almost as much as the group which had actually practiced. This particular study showed that *mental imaging* can improve one's ability to shoot basketball free throws. The same technique has been successfully used for improving one's golf game, tennis game, and other sports.

By adding training motions to the technique of mental imaging, you can train your muscles and your mind to improve your performance. Mental imaging by itself will imprint the subconscious, but adding the physical training motions will train the muscles to repeat the same successful sports moves over and over again with more endurance.

Mental and Physical Imaging

Let's suppose you want to apply Synergetics Imaging to improving your golf game. You play once a week on your day off, and sometimes twice, but you aren't getting in enough strokes to keep your muscles and your mind working together for a grooved swing. At the most you are swinging at the ball maybe a couple of hundred times a week.

Now, let's play a golf game with Synergetics Imaging:

- Place a golf ball on the carpet in front of you, right where it would be for whichever club you decide to practice with.

- Reach into your imaginary golf bag, pull out your imaginary club, and address the ball, hooking your fingers together and pulling with good resistance.

- Slowly pull into your backswing (you'll notice the motion is almost identical to the Extended Low Pull) very slowly, with good steady resistance, but not so much that your hands or arms quiver.

- Hesitate for a couple of counts at the top of your backswing, then very slowly with strong control swing down "through the ball," follow through, and hold your follow-through for a couple of counts with your head down and your eyes still riveted on the golf ball (or on the imaginary spot where you placed the imaginary golf ball if you didn't have a real one handy).

- After a couple of counts, raise your head and "watch" the golf ball arch its way to a perfect landing in the middle of the fairway or on the green, at just the right distance (depending on the imaginary club you chose). If you know your course, then play each hole as if you were actually there.

- Also practice a series of swings with the Rainbow Extended Low Push to develop more control over the rest of your "swing" muscles.

In 12 minutes, you can slowly, with conscious control, swing 120 to 180 times at the ball (more than if you had played twenty-seven holes of golf). Use different imaginary clubs, adjusting your position to the ball, and imagining the fairway, the green, the tee, and the shot. Play as many imaginary rounds as you feel like. If you practiced Synergetics Imaging for just 12 minutes, once a day, you would be getting in the equivalent practice strokes of about ten or fifteen practice rounds of golf a week. You should experience more power, control, and flexibility the next time you take your real clubs out of the bag and swing at the ball. You would also be getting a great physical workout for your general health.

Although we used the example of how Synergetics Imaging can work for improving your golf game, it can be applied to any sport or physical activity that you want to improve on. For example, modify the Rainbow Series to duplicate some of your tennis strokes. Change your body position, get down "low on the ball," follow through, keep your head fixed on the ideal spot for your imaginary ball as you go through the stroke, or even hang a tennis ball in front of you. The Extended Chest-High Pull and Push can help train your body for more powerful forehands and backhands. The Grip Twist, Grip Switch, The Hook, and The Rooster will add strength and control to your wrists and forearms for tennis. The same goes for football, basketball, racquetball, baseball, soccer. Use your imagination to modify the Synergetics motions to fit your training program.

WARM UP!

Over the years the *warm-up* has changed dramatically. When I played college football back in the late forties the pregame warm-ups were more like a full scale scrimmage. Many of us were exhausted before we lined up for the kickoff! Now the warm-ups look more like a ballet class—stretching, slowly moving legs and arms to their maximum stretch, sometimes with the help of a teammate. After a little running around, the game begins. Eleven players from each squad battle each other on the field while the other thirty or so players on each team sit on the bench, growing stiff and cold. No wonder there are so many injuries in sports today! A player should not enter a game of any kind without first warming up the body to playing level.

Unfortunately, in many competitive sports, the coaches do not give the players time to warm up before they are sent off the bench into the game. But there is no reason that you can't give your body a good warm-up before you get into your game. *Don't be self-conscious about warming up.* Here's how you can cut your soreness, injuries, and your losses.

Since Synergetics combines stretching, strength exercise, and aerobics in one motion, you can get all the warm-up you need with a series of Rainbows, Stepping Out Pluses, and Cat Stretches. Do a minimum of 5 of each Basic Rainbow (Pulls and Pushes) at the Basic Tempo, and if time permits, a series of 5 of each Extended Rainbow (Pulls and Pushes) at Breezing Tempo. Finish off your warm-up with a minimum of 20 Stepping Out Pluses right and left and a series of 40 Cat Stretches. Accentuate your Power Breathing with every flex. Then pace back and forth for a couple of minutes, still Power Breathing, concentrating on your body and your upcoming game. Your blood is pumping at game levels, and all of your muscles are tuned for the action. Now you're ready to win!

The game is over. You played well! Now cool down with some slow, gentle Synergetics of your choice to realign your body and dissipate the acid byproducts of metabolism that have built up in your muscles while you were playing. Tonight you will sleep more soundly, and tomorrow morning you will wake up feeling better than you ever have after a physical competition. The habit of warming up and cooling down with Synergetics will add years to your playing career.

THE ULTIMATE ATHLETE

An All Pro football player? A Hall of Fame basketball player? A bonus baseball pitcher? No, you! You can be an ultimate athlete in your own right—regardless of your age! By our definition, the ultimate athlete is one who develops all of his or her natural physical abilities—not necessarily for games or sports, but for everyday life. Even though you may never be required to use an above average amount of physical strength and quickness, it is important that you always have it in reserve. There may be a time when you will need the power and agility to save someone's life, or maybe your own. Thousands of people are severely injured every year in household accidents and playing weekend sports—many of which could have been avoided if the person involved had possessed an athletic body.

An athletic body is a beautiful body; it comes in all shapes and sizes, and all ages. The athletic body moves with grace instead of lurching as it walks. The athletic body carries itself tall, with an inner strength and pride. The athletic body is full of energy and radiance. The athletic body accomplishes a great deal in its life—enjoying every minute of it. The athletic body makes you turn around and admire it. Mother Nature gave us all the potential to possess an athletic body, and she gave us all the power and the ability to regenerate ourselves at any point in our lives if we choose.

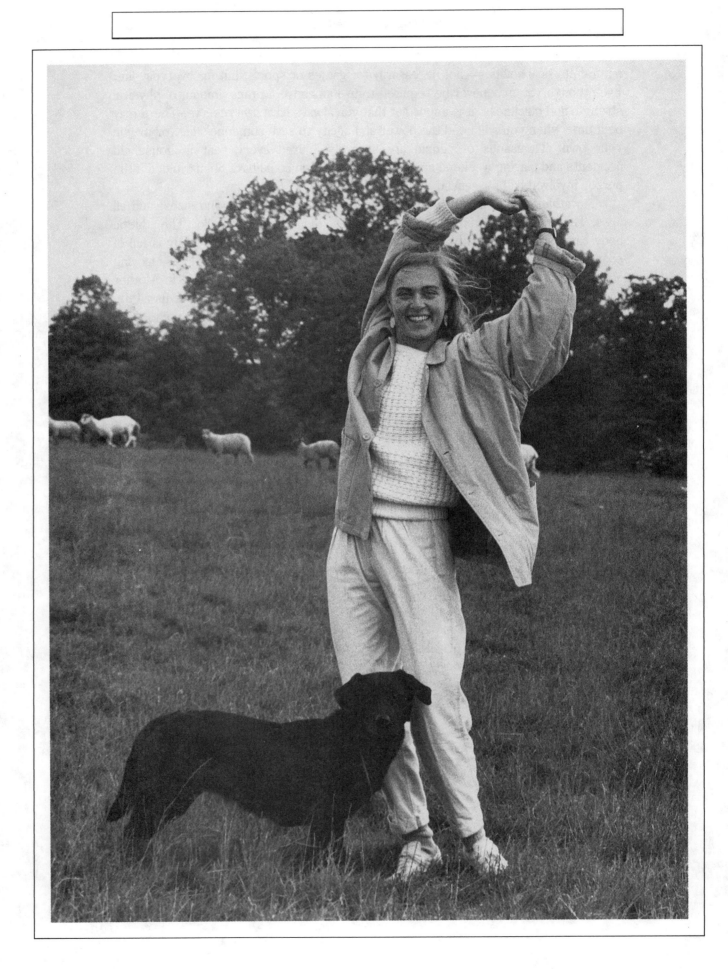

14

The Choice
Is Yours

Once I asked a friend why he was working so hard. He answered that he was earning the money to "buy himself some options." This word, *options,* didn't mean much to me until I looked it up in a dictionary. Option means freedom of choice. What my friend was telling me is that he wanted enough money so he would be free to do whatever he pleased, when he pleased, and how he pleased. But, is it really a lot of money that gives us freedom of choice? I don't think so.

I think our options are only limited by the energy we have, and that we often don't have the energy to do all of the things that we would like to do. I remember when I first started writing this book, I didn't think I would ever have enough time or energy to finish it. After all, I was running a real estate company and helping raise a big family, wasn't I?

So, I started training myself like an athlete—going to bed at a reasonable hour, carefully choosing the foods I knew I should eat, and of course, exercising like I said everyone else should.

In time I was able to gather the energy and the will to write instead of just sitting around wasting my time, fretting and wishing. After a while, I began to create a work habit that I had never had before in my life. I was able to sit down and get things done because I wanted to, not because I had to. Instead of talking about writing, I was doing it. I was putting my typewriter where my mouth was. I was experiencing a new-found freedom of choice for myself that just a year before had been a dream that would never come true. That was the beginning of my new life— a life where I can do more of what I choose to do.

What choices do you want to have in your life? Have you got the strength and energy to go after them? Are you willing to pay the price in time and energy to do something that you have been wishing to do all of your life, but keep putting off over and over again? I want to learn how to play good country guitar, learn how to speak Spanish, and learn to write novels. What would you like to do in your life that you haven't done yet? Do you feel that you are too busy just surviving to take on any more activities?

Somewhere back in time, a primitive hunter returned to his cave-home bearing food from his day of hunting. After sharing the evening meal with his family, he quietly reached into the crackling fire where they huddled and withdrew a flaming piece of wood. Then, holding his torch high over his head, he went deeper into the darkness of the cavern. That night, with his torch held smoldering in the crack of a rock to light his work, he scratched the crude outline of the bison that he hunted by day on the dimly lit wall of his cave. He had chosen to draw a picture of an animal on that stone wall not because he had to, but because he wanted to—because he had the energy to do more than just roll over and go to sleep until another day of "surviving" dawned. Little did he know that someday his anonymous art would be famous throughout the world.

Someone once said, "You've got to be in love to want to stay in shape." We truly believe that. We have to be in love with life to want to take care of ourselves. We must have conscious, strong reasons to want to live a long, healthy life. We must find things that we freely choose to keep us excited, so that we can't wait to bound out of bed in the morning to get at them. I remember thinking that I was too old to begin writing—that most writers started when they were young, and had to write for years before they could do anything of value. I also thought that when people reached a certain age, their life should start winding down. I thought that we had to look and act a certain way when we reached a certain age. Then the truth slowly dawned on me. I had been blindly following the teachings and examples of all of those poor souls who had completely given up on their own lives.

We have a new life every day if we take the time and energy to care for ourselves. And regardless of our age, condition, or situation, we can do as well as that simple, yet artistic hunter of the past, who drew his primitive animal picture on the dark wall of that cave many thousands of years ago—because he *wanted to*.

I am approaching sixty years old as I write this sentence, and my life has truly just begun because of the energy I have. Joanna and I hope that Synergetics will be your first, best step to energy that will lead you to your treasure of options. This is your great beginning, your life can be exciting and full of goodness every day, as you make your own free choices, and care for your own perfect body.

To Your Health and Your Happiness,

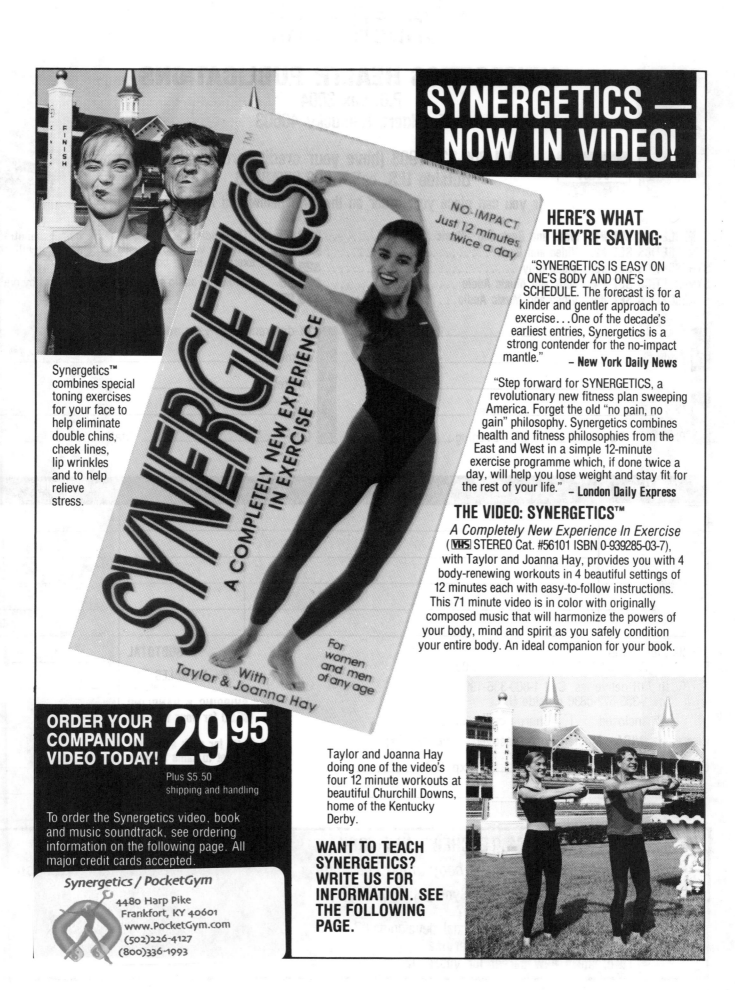

MasterCard

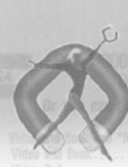

RICAN PRESS

DISCOVER

SYNERGETICS
SYNERGETICS
SYNERGETICS
SYNERGETICS
SYNERGETICS

SOLD TO

Your Na
Address

City
Phone

min. music soundtrack
in conjunction with the

is companions by mail.

te_____ Zip_____

How Many		Extended Price

SPECIAL HAN
For C.O.D. A

For Rush Al
(or 1

☐ Check e

Circle one:

Credit Card

Signature _

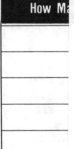